Modeling the Injury Flow and Treatment after Major Earthquakes

AF729453

Lulu Zhang
Editor

Modeling the Injury Flow and Treatment after Major Earthquakes

Springer

Editor
Lulu Zhang
Department of Military Health Service
College of Military Health Service
Second Military Medical University
Shanghai
China

The research was supported by the major project in the '12th Five-Year Plan' of the People's Liberation Army (LZ grant number: AWS12J002), the major program of National Nature Science Foundation Project of China (LZ grant number: 71233008), the joint research project of major diseases of Shanghai health system (LZ grant number: 2013ZYJB0006), and the National Natural Science Foundation of China (LZ grant number: 91224005, YL grant number: 71573270, XL grant number: 71303249), the "Morning Project" of Shanghai Education Committee (XL grant number 13CG41)

ISBN 978-94-024-1370-0 ISBN 978-94-017-7527-4 (eBook)
DOI 10.1007/978-94-017-7527-4

Springer Dordrecht Heidelberg New York London
© Springer Science+Business Media Dordrecht 2016
Softcover reprint of the hardcover 1st edition 2016
This work is subject to copyright. All rights are reserved by the Publisher, whether the whole or part of the material is concerned, specifically the rights of translation, reprinting, reuse of illustrations, recitation, broadcasting, reproduction on microfilms or in any other physical way, and transmission or information storage and retrieval, electronic adaptation, computer software, or by similar or dissimilar methodology now known or hereafter developed.
The use of general descriptive names, registered names, trademarks, service marks, etc. in this publication does not imply, even in the absence of a specific statement, that such names are exempt from the relevant protective laws and regulations and therefore free for general use.
The publisher, the authors and the editors are safe to assume that the advice and information in this book are believed to be true and accurate at the date of publication. Neither the publisher nor the authors or the editors give a warranty, express or implied, with respect to the material contained herein or for any errors or omissions that may have been made.

Printed on acid-free paper

Springer Science+Business Media B.V. Dordrecht is part of Springer Science+Business Media (www.springer.com)

Contents

Chapter 1
Introduction

Bihan Tang and Lulu Zhang

Abstract Earthquakes have a devastating impact on affected regions and their populations, often causing death and serious personal injury. They often result in incalculable environmental damage, loss of life, and threats to health. China is an earthquake-prone country located at the intersection of the circum-Pacific seismic zone and the Eurasian seismic zone. After the Wenchuan earthquake, China began to build an emergency medical rescue system for natural disasters. Tremendous progress has been made in response to many medical challenges resulting from these disasters. However, emergency medical rescue is complicated, and substantial emphasis should be placed on its organization to achieve optimal results. Further studies should focus on medical rescue efforts in terms of emergency response, collaboration and cooperation, large-scale transportation and rehabilitation of sick and wounded people, the public health response, and the effect on mental health and social institutions.

1.1 Background

1.1.1 Medical Relief System in China

1.1.1.1 System and Status of Chinese Earthquake Emergency Rescue Work

Chinese earthquake emergency rescue work began following the 1966 Xingtai earthquake. It has undergone multiple stages, such as establishment of the concept of earthquake emergency formation, proposition of earthquake emergency

B. Tang
Department of Military Health Service, College of Military Health Service,
Second Military Medical University, Yangpu, Shanghai, China
e-mail: mangotangbihan@126.com

L. Zhang (✉)
Department of Military Health Service, College of Military Health Service,
Second Military Medical University, Shanghai, China
e-mail: zllrmit@aliyun.com

© Springer Science+Business Media Dordrecht 2016
L. Zhang (ed.), *Modeling the Injury Flow and Treatment after Major Earthquakes*, DOI 10.1007/978-94-017-7527-4_1

measures, legalization of earthquake emergency rescue, and systematization of earthquake emergency work. Now, there exists an earthquake emergency response system and operation mechanism with a unified government under the leadership of the earthquake comprehensive coordination departments at all levels, the division responsible for the relevant departments, in which the general population, the military, and the police all participate. The established earthquake emergency rescue system is supported by laws and regulations and based on contingency plans. The core technology is an emergency command structure that is supported by the emergency response platform, with an emergency rescue team as the backbone and emergency equipment and materials as the protection.[1]

In China, especially after major emergencies, the State Council, as a chief leading organization of national emergency management, usually coordinates the relationships between various departments of the State Council by establishing or initiating permanent or temporary agency headquarters. For example, the State established the "earthquake relief headquarters" after the Wenchuan earthquake. Meanwhile, the General Office of the State Council also set up the State Emergency Management Office to undertake comprehensive emergency management coordination responsibilities. According to the notification of deliberation and coordination mechanism by State Council (Guo Fa [2008] No. 13), the State Council earthquake relief headquarters is the coordinating agency in the State for procedures in the sequence of specific work by State institutions, which is undertaken by the China Seismological Bureau.

As a coordinating body for procedures, the State Council earthquake relief headquarters does not establish substantive offices—it currently only establishes the Office of the State Council Earthquake Relief Headquarters in the State Seismological Bureau. Only after the earthquake and after approval from the State Council is the usual joint meeting of the leadership of the State Council earthquake disaster reduction and dispatching earthquake disaster reduction transferred to the earthquake relief headquarters of the State Council, which is responsible for earthquake disaster and emergency relief work (Zhang et al. 2012).

In the earthquake emergency rescue process, in accordance with the earthquake "national earthquake emergency plan," governments and departments at all levels bear their respective earthquake emergency command tasks in response to the grading requirements. Among them, level I emergency response occurs after a major earthquake, enacted specifically by the People's Government leaders of the affected areas of the province (autonomous regions and municipalities), as well as the State Council earthquake relief headquarters unified organizational leadership, with direction and coordination of the national earthquake emergency work headed by the State Council leaders. Level II emergency response occurs after a major earthquake and is enacted by the People's Government leaders of the affected areas of the province (autonomous regions and municipalities); the China Seismological

[1] Gao Xing, Emergency mechanism for medical assistance in May 12 Wenchuan earthquake [J], CHINA JOURNAL OF EMERGENCY RESUSCITATION AND DISASTER MEDICINE, Vol.3, No.6

Bureau, under the leadership of the State Council, is responsible for organizing and coordinating national earthquake emergency work. Level III emergency response occurs after a major earthquake and is enacted by the People's Government leaders of the affected areas of the city (prefecture, league); the China Seismological Bureau organizes and coordinates the work of the national earthquake emergency, and the Deputy Secretary is in charge of the China Seismological Bureau. Level IV emergency response occurs after a general earthquake and is enacted by the People's Government leaders of the affected areas of the province (autonomous regions and municipalities) and the Municipal People's Government (prefecture, league). Earthquake emergency work is implemented under the support of People's Government leadership and the county disaster area (city, district, and flag). The China Seismological Bureau organizes and coordinates the work of the national earthquake emergency, and the Deputy Secretary is in charge of the China Seismological Bureau (Zhang et al. 2011).

1.1.1.2 Effectiveness and Issues with Chinese Earthquake Emergency Rescue System

After 40 years of efforts, China's earthquake emergency rescue work has made considerable progress. Particularly in the first decade of the twenty-first century, earthquake emergency rescue work, as one of the three working earthquake disaster mitigation systems, has achieved rapid development. It effectively responded to the 2008 Wenchuan earthquake and the 2010 Yushu earthquake; however, some problems and shortcomings were also exposed. Practice is the sole criterion for testing truth. The Wenchuan and Yushu earthquakes were two major challenges of China's ability to deal with unexpected disasters. They also allow for comprehensive examination of the effectiveness of the earthquake emergency rescue system.

Rapid Earthquake Response

The sudden and devastating traits of earthquake disasters, especially major earthquake disasters, determine the importance of timing in earthquake emergency rescue, which is the key to reducing casualties and economic losses. Fast earthquake disaster response depends primarily on whether the acquisition is timely and the decision is scientific. The China Seismological Bureau made a quick report and initiated level I response 13 min after the Wenchuan earthquake. Then, the State Council established earthquake relief headquarters more than 1 h after the disaster. The China Seismological Bureau made a quick report and initiated level II (after 1 h, it was changed to level I) response 11 min after the Wenchuan earthquake. Then, the State Council established an earthquake relief headquarters no more than 1 h after the disaster. The response to these two earthquakes was relatively quick and timely, but that to the Yushu earthquake was faster (Kang et al. 2012).

It is undeniable, however, that there remains room for improvement in Chinese earthquake emergency response, and the key is that the disaster information must be continuous, accurate, and dynamic. Although Chinese authorities have established the appropriate seismic monitoring system to carry out work related to forecasting and early warning of disaster risk, the utilization of disaster risk information, analysis, evaluation, and forecasting is inadequate; the risk evaluation index system is imperfect, which is not conducive to comprehensive mitigation and early warning. During the Wenchuan earthquake, the access to disaster information was singular and backward, and the disaster quick report network failed to play its intended role. The communication system was affected by large-scale paralysis, blocking submission of the disaster information, and information of severe damage in Beichuan County was received 24 h after the disaster. Further, China lacks a forecasting system for seismic intensity and satellite, aerial reconnaissance means, which seriously affected the policy-making departments in the ability to make prompt and accurate determinations during the disaster. After 2 years, during the Yushu earthquake, the progress of information techniques and the application of satellite remote-sensing technology enhance the speed and accuracy of disaster information acquisition. However, it cannot fully meet the needs of emergency rescue, and as a result, receiving disaster information quickly and accurately to facilitate quick response in the earthquake remains an important issue.

Professional Rescue Force

A major earthquake can release tremendous energy in a moment, resulting in many buildings collapsing. Meanwhile, it may bring about many secondary disasters, resulting in greater difficulties in disaster rescue work. Obviously, the rescue task cannot be competent without multifaceted rescue forces in considerable quantity and quality. Over the years, China has established a professional rescue team of more than 50 million people to deal with a variety of unexpected disasters, which has played a critical role in emergency rescue during earthquakes, floods, landslides, fires, mining accidents, hazardous chemical explosions, and other disasters. Although the formation time of the professional rescue time is rather short, it has become the elite troop in the previous earthquake relief work with its advanced concepts, high-quality skills, and professional equipment. The Wenchuan earthquake was one of the largest tests for our professional rescue forces. China devoted up to 2.6 million professional rescue people to the Wenchuan earthquake, including 20 national and provincial earthquake disaster emergency rescue teams, 41 mine rescue teams, and 29 fire brigades, all of whom engaged in difficult tasks, successfully rescuing 7439 survivors buried under the ruins. During the Yushu earthquake, nine national and provincial earthquake disaster emergency rescue teams rushed to the disaster area, and their equipment level and rescue efficiency all had improved relative to the Wenchuan emergency relief, but overall, China's major professional rescue forces still cannot meet the needs of earthquake disaster emergency rescue. First, most professional rescue teams still lack specialized rescue training, earthquake relief equipment, and field experience. Second, the total quantity of seismic specialized rescue teams remains inadequate, and they cannot reach the initial disaster areas, let alone launch a massive search and rescue for a large number of buried people in major disasters. Third, it remains unsatisfactory for conducting rescues under mountain plateaus and in poisonous circumstances. Further, there remain gaps in our earthquake relief efforts compared with developed countries. Professional rescuers only accounted for 3 % of the total population, and the percentage is even smaller in the western seismogenic zone. The level of technical equipment and training of various professional rescue forces cannot meet modern complex rescue needs under difficult conditions. Therefore, further expansion of the earthquake professional rescue teams and strengthened professional rescue forces of earthquake drills are imperative.

People's Self-Aid and Mutual Aid

In earthquakes, the general public in addition to emergency rescuers themselves are the direct victims of emergency rescue. We can say that people's self-help and mutual aid is the first form of earthquake disaster emergency rescue at the scene. Practice at home and abroad shows that, in the majority of earthquake disasters, many lives are saved from self-help and mutual aid. In the Tangshan earthquake of 1976, 86 % (about 60 million) of the citizens were buried in the ruins. Among them, about 48 million people were saved by self-help and mutual aid from the disaster grassroots organizations and common people. In the Wenchuan earthquake of 2008, survivors who were saved by self-help and mutual aid made up 80 % of the total survivors. Thus, in the golden time after an earthquake, the stricken areas in particular are isolated from the outside world, and public awareness of self-help and mutual aid and the degree of organization are of crucial significance for removing individuals from danger and saving lives. According to statistics, 20 min after an earthquake, buried people are rescued at a 98 % success rate, which drops to 63 % 1 h after the earthquake. Among those who had not been rescued with 2 h after an earthquake, 58 % died of suffocation (Kang et al. 2012). Thus, self-help and mutual aid is the quickest and most effective method to alleviate casualties, as rescue between neighbors is fastest, most convenient in space, and most familiar in terms of living environment. In developing countries, mobilizing people to actively participate in rescue to fully engage community relief organizations is a major feature and highlight of emergency disaster management. In China, information on earthquake disaster reduction is inadequately disseminated. There is a lack of education regarding society-wide risk prevention and emergency management disposal and specific requirements for training and drill measures that are in place are unclear. Especially in vast rural and small-town areas, earthquake emergency training is generally lacking, and people's awareness of their own social crisis, risk awareness, and first-aid knowledge and skills are very weak, professional representation is poor, and unawareness is large. These factors together result in weak earthquake disaster prevention and practical ability. Above all, recruiting the public, implementing earthquake preparedness at the grassroots level, establishing rescue volunteers, and active engagement in first-aid skills training are vital to minimizing casualties after earthquakes.

Earthquake Emergency Plan

Preparedness ensures success and unpreparedness spells failure. The earthquake emergency plan is the basis of the work carried out during earthquake emergencies, including emergency action guidelines and an emergency command program. Inner and outer earthquake disaster mitigation shows that establishing a sound scientific and practical contingency plan is the basic necessity for efficient and orderly enactment of earthquake emergency rescue and an important safeguard in reducing the impact of earthquake disasters. In early 1988, we began to advance formulations of contingency plans in some earthquake surveillance and protection zones and have formed a national earthquake emergency plan that combines vertical and horizontal systems, which has played an important role in previous earthquake disaster emergency rescues. In the Wenchuan earthquake, the State Council and local governments at all levels and relevant departments quickly activate contingency plans, form various types of command structure, carry out emergency relief operations effectively, and ensure the order and efficiency of the relief work. Those schools, hospitals, and stadiums that emphasize earthquake emergency plan exercises usually respond rapidly at the time of the earthquake, greatly reducing casualties. As handling of the Yushu earthquake was informed by lessons learned during the Wenchuan earthquake, its emergency plan was more comprehensive, which played an important role in organization of various emergency resources, rescue and recovery work in production, and living order. Overall, however, there are still significant deficiencies in the pertinence, coordination, and comprehensiveness of the Chinese earthquake emergency plan. First, there are significant deficiencies in the earthquake catastrophe system, as it lacks specific disaster grading and corresponding measures. The command system and operation mechanism could not adapt to disaster emergency needs for the Wenchuan earthquake. Second, existing types of emergency plans at all levels lack interrelationships across different levels and departments, and the headquarters lacks plan-level responsibility constraints. Third, preplanning does not contain enough comprehensive elements, and various rescue forces and volunteers across regional organizations are not included in coordination and management. After Wenchuan, the Yushu earthquake emergency plan with regard to preparation and revision of all localities and departments has been put on the agenda. In the future, we must accelerate progress and improve the mechanism to establish a dynamic and continuously improving emergency plan for combat and maneuverability.

1.1.2 Significance of China's Medical Relief Effort from Earthquakes

1.1.2.1 Worldwide Earthquakes as a Frequent Threat to Human Life and Property Safety

Earthquakes are natural phenomena, but they also cause a great deal of harm given the force of natural disasters. Earthquakes cause seismic ground shaking through shock waves, resulting in damage and collapse of buildings, roads, and bridges,

Table 1.1 Public safety requirements for emergency rescue

Disaster type	Pre-alarm or emergency time	Occurrence season	Occurrence location
Floods	Several days to 10 days of warning time	Rainy season	River basin
Landslides, mudslides	Hours to days of continuous rainfall	Rainy season	Mountains
Typhoons	1 week to 10 days of warning time	Summer	Along the sea
Forest fire	Several hours	Dry season	Forest zone
Earthquakes	Usually zero	Year round	Nationwide
Fire	Usually zero, predictable prone points	Year round	Place with people
Public health	Zero to dozens of days	Year round	Nationwide
Production safety	Zero	Year round	Productive place

breaking and tilting of the ground, landslides, debris flow, and tsunamis. Meanwhile, due to the damage to buildings after earthquakes, they also result in fire, flammable gas leaks, damaged nuclear facilities and nuclear leaks, and other secondary disasters. China is located in two seismic zones—the intersecting parts of the circum-Pacific seismic belt and the Eurasian seismic zone with high frequency of seismic activity, high strength, light source, and wide distribution. Accordingly, China is frequently hit by earthquakes. In 2008, an 8.0 earthquake on the Richter scale occurred in Sichuan, China, causing 6.9 million deaths and 37.6 million people injured, resulting in the most casualties since the Tangshan earthquake (Kang et al. 2012). In less than 2 years, on April 14, 2010, a 7.1 magnitude earthquake occurred in the Tibetan Autonomous Prefecture of Yushu region, ultimately resulting in 2698 deaths and 12,135 people injured. Earthquakes appear to have become an unconventional social emergency that threatens human life and property safety.

Due to its vast and complex geological features, China has always been a highly earthquake-affected country. Earthquake disasters are frequent and high in strength, resulting in heavy casualties and widespread features. In the twentieth century, the total number of global deaths due to earthquakes is nearly 1.2 million, of which China accounts for nearly half (600,000). From 1949 to 2000, the number of deaths caused by natural disasters of all kinds was about 550,000, while earthquakes caused more than half of these (about 280,000). The Chinese earthquake death toll is the highest in the world, ranking first among all kinds of natural disasters.

We can see from Table 1.1 that the emergency rapid response capability for earthquakes is the most difficult. With the advent of the information age, post-earthquake emergency response situations for devastating earthquakes (e.g., 2008 Wenchuan earthquake, Yushu earthquake) are always amplified by the media. In emergency response work, response speed of the relevant emergency departments and the quality of multi-sectored coordination between emergency rescue workers not only play an important role in the success of disaster response but also can easily become the focus of public questioning. Therefore, our study on responses to devastating earthquake emergencies is of substantial research value.

1.1.2.2 Earthquake Emergency Medical Rescue Law and Establishing a Scientific Rescue System

Scientific research on rules for earthquake emergency medical rescue contributes to the accumulation of valuable experience in the practice of medical rescue following earthquake emergencies, promotes proper function of the health emergency system and working mechanism, and scientifically improves the national emergency medical rescue capabilities. Since the event of “atypical pneumonia,” the Chinese government has continued to accumulate emergency medical rescue practice from public health emergencies and natural disasters. Over the past decade, health emergency departments have conducted extensive research, teaching, and training on public health emergencies and natural disaster emergency medical rescue issues.

After the Wenchuan earthquake, the Chinese government profoundly summarized and reflected on earthquake emergency medical relief operations and conducted extensive research and capacity building on emergency organization and command, rescue forces and deployment pumping groups, and casualty treatment and evacuation (Zhang et al. 2011). However, comprehensive and systematic research at the national level for natural disaster relief medicine is lacking, which leads to serious deficiencies in the accumulation and consolidation of valuable experience. Consequently, efficient emergency medical rescue operations for disaster relief remain insufficient. Thus, the Chinese health emergency system should transfer from the “framework” of a gradual transition to a “standardized management” stage as soon as possible, expand extensive research on public health emergencies and natural disasters emergency medical problems, and seek to grasp the special rules under the particular background of “emergency medical rescue.” This work presents a higher health emergency requirement: we should implement quality control and performance management thinking in every action, including the development of plans of action to carry out, inspect, and evaluate by implementing gradual adjustment. Our study is not only a summary and retrospective analysis of pre-natural medical disaster relief work but also an accumulation and exploration of evaluation system establishment, which will provide a reference on methods and paths of emergency medical aid for future work.

1.1.2.3 Modeling of Earthquake Emergency Medical Rescue and Improvement of Rescue Efficiency

Through empirical analysis of the earthquake emergency medical discoveries, we can see that the “two phases” of earthquake casualties (i.e., the growth phase and stable phase) and “three-stage” feature of rescue operations (i.e., emergency period, effective period, and maintenance period) constitute a general law of earthquake emergency medical rescue. Conducting seismic emergency medical rescue organization and command, power organization and management, task switching, and power construction according to this law can help improve the efficiency of earthquake emergency medical rescue. Research on earthquake casualties that occur is essential for improving earthquake emergency medical rescue. According to the investigation of the reported death toll in various earthquakes domestically and abroad, we found that the reported death toll is associated with timing of deaths. Rescue personnel rescue those who are trapped in the rubble, need to clean, find, rescue survivors in every house, and simultaneously conduct the search for victims. Therefore, the number of deaths and injuries has a good correlation with the curves presented by their reported time, respectively. More deaths reflect an increased amount of time to rescue the buried and later time to quoted time. The later the rate of casualties stabilized, the more inadequate the disaster aid and the longer the issue will be extended. Practice at home and abroad shows that the survival rate is high in early rescue with a sharp decline in the survival rate of later rescue. Through a review analysis of several earthquakes, we found that survival rate is a function of the wounded after tune of the earthquake. The inflection point of the two phases of earthquake casualties is related to the elements such as earthquake scale and location; as a result, forecasting the inflection point of earthquake casualties with relevant data is highly important to earthquake emergency medical relief organization decisions, especially in the use of power, medical evacuation, and so on.

1.2 Study Design and System Thinking

China is an earthquake-prone country located in the intersection area of the circum-Pacific seismic belt and the Eurasian seismic zone. In recent years, the 2008 Wenchuan earthquake and the 2010 Yushu earthquake caused a considerable number of deaths, health deficits, and environmental damage. The Chinese health system is in need of theoretical guidance on emergency medical relief. Although medical science has undergone substantial development, disaster medicine has not received enough attention. Major disaster relief always permits acquisition of valuable experience and lessons to be learned, which was gained only through the blood and lives of millions of victims and rescue workers. Emergency medical rescue relief is an extremely complex system to engineer. The problem of emergency medical rescue relief is extremely complex, involving a wide range, such as the occurrence of earthquake casualties, medical evacuation, allocation of medical rescue forces, organization and command of earthquake rescue forces, location and distribution of medical rescue institutions, and so on. Whether effective coping mechanisms and plans for a variety of disasters are established will directly affect the speed, capacity, and efficiency of the emergency medical rescue. Speed is not a substitute for efficiency, and improving efficiency must rely on the scientific method, relying on theoretical research support. Thus, it is essential to establish a corresponding model to support the improvement of the disaster rescue system.

1.2.1 Study Design and Technology Roadmap

This book applied numerous modeling methods to analyze in detail the occurrence of earthquake casualties, hospital length of stay, medical evacuation, medical rescue force allocation, organization and command of earthquake rescue forces, location and distribution of medical support institutions, peacetime to wartime in hospitals, and so on. This book aims to find the intervention targets of earthquake rescue through simulation and modeling intervention, thus effectively improving rescue efficiency and providing a theoretical basis for future rescue capabilities.

1.2.2 Previous Research

Our investigation group began following the 2008 "5.12" Wenchuan earthquake, focusing on earthquake emergency medical rescue operations (Zhang et al. 2012). We went deep into earthquake-stricken areas for data collection and field research and completed the *Wenchuan Earthquake Relief Medical Service Investigation Report*, which was published in the *Liberation Army Daily Internal Reference*. After the 2010 "4.14" earthquake in Yushu, Qinghai Province, we assumed the Ministry of Health (now the State Planning Commission Guardian)'s mandatory subject task project, "Yushu earthquake emergency medical rescue external evaluation," and sent the investigation team to earthquake-stricken areas for on-site research and data collection. Based on the "two main lines," wounded flow and rescue forces, we launched systematic research from three levels: strategic, operational, and disastrous. We focused on casualties, on-site treatment, medical evacuation, hospital treatment, epidemic prevention, and psychological rescue, which refer to "wounded" as the main line. Further, we focused on rescue forces and deployment, structure, organization and command, and allocative efficiency, which refer to "rescue forces" as the main line of content. We submitted *Chinese Qinghai Yushu earthquake relief medicine evaluation report* to the Ministry of Health and published *An Empirical Study of Earthquake Medical Rescue* (Science Press). In 2013, Sichuan Province underwent another earthquake, "4.20" Lushan earthquake. We went to the disaster area 3 months after the event for investigation. Compared to the previous two investigations, the focus of this study was more forward and covered the IX intensity stricken areas in depth. We constructed a large-scale questionnaire study for earthquake-hit residents, focusing on earthquake relief reactivity and accessibility. This investigation covered the two most severely stricken towns, distributing 6200 questionnaires and recycling 5800 questionnaires. During the same time, we launched an investigation among different levels of rescue personnel about their behavior and studied earthquake-related relief and rescue needs.

1.2.3 Aims and Objectives of the Project

1.2.3.1 Objectives of the Project

Since the emergency rescue studies on the 2008 earthquake, our group has sustained attention on the three major earthquakes of Wenchuan, Yushu, and Lushan, accumulating a great deal of valuable experience and background data. To find the key technologies of earthquake emergency rescue, this book focuses on the modeling, simulation, and policy intervention of injury flow and its rescue process. It fills gaps in the field of international medical relief in disaster response modeling and provides valuable guidance and reference for the practice of medicine and theoretical study of disaster relief. This book is designed mainly for professionals in the field of international health emergency rescue and provides scientific policy support and informative experience for the international medical rescue earthquake emergency rescue and provides strong technical support for emergency operations related to international disaster relief agencies.

The book consists of seven parts. The first is a general section (Chap. 1), mainly outlining the background of the study, the purpose and significance of the data sources, and describing the method of system dynamics and its related principles. The second part (Chaps. 2, 3, 4, 5, 6, 7, and 8) covers models on the occurrence of earthquake casualties, the length of stay among hospitalized patients, medical evacuation after earthquakes, medical rescue force allocation after earthquakes, organization and command of earthquake rescue forces, location and distribution of medical rescue institutions, and from peacetime to wartime in hospital. Each chapter includes an introduction to the casualty data, data source, construction of the conceptual model, logical model and SD model, reality simulation, modeling intervention, and a summary. The third part (Chap. 9) summarizes and provides scientific policy recommendations according to the results of our modeling and simulation.

1.2.3.2 Project Objectives

To further improve and perfect health emergency system and its working mechanism and to provide policy recommendations for international emergency rescue, the research group members have been to Wenchuan, the Ministry of Health, Yushu in Qinghai Province, Lushan, and other places in Sichuan for earthquake emergency medical rescue scene investigation. Based on large-scale field research and data collection, we scientifically evaluated the occurrence of earthquake casualties, the length of stay among hospitalized patients, medical evacuation after earthquakes, medical rescue force allocation after earthquakes, the organization and command of earthquake rescue forces, and location and distribution of medical support institutions through scientific analysis and systemic evaluation, elucidating the earthquake medical rescue experience and summarizing the Chinese earthquake relief efforts and policy intervention targets. The book focuses on systemic research of Chinese earthquake disaster emergency medical rescue operations, summarizing valuable experience with earthquake disaster emergency medical rescue to establish the occurrence and treatment of the background of wounded streaming data, systematically and comprehensively proposing earthquake rescue methodology, and forming a theoretical earthquake emergency rescue framework model. Accordingly, we established a decision support platform to assess the efficiency of rescue forces configured with scientific thinking and advanced theoretical methods. Our study has produced valuable knowledge for international natural disaster emergency relief work and complements international disaster emergency intervention model building and policy gap simulation, which has far-reaching significance.

1.2.4 Data Resource and Collection

1.2.4.1 Existing Data Collection

1. Relevant documents issued by the National Ministry of Health
2. Duty information from the National Ministry of Health
3. The overall condition of medical health workers and the vehicle sent during the Qinghai Yushu earthquake
4. Information tables reported by the National Ministry of Health
5. Information statistics from health and epidemic prevention work group
6. Meeting abstract of the health emergency leading group from the Yushu Ministry of Health in Qinghai Province
7. Information table of reconstruction
8. Epidemic report of material dispatching

1.2.4.2 On-Site Research Data

According to the evaluation plan of our research group, we went to Sichuan and Qinghai Provinces for emergency medical rescue field investigation. Our research mainly focused on "three levels," "two lines," and "three kinds of objects," that is, local rescue forces, regional support, and strategy support force; the "wounded flow" of injury, treatment, and prevention of mental evacuation and "rescue forces" command and force deployment; command structure, rescue squad, and rescue personnel (Gautschi et al. 2008).

Our investigation data contain the following: (1) the occurrence of casualties during earthquakes; (2) investigation of headquarters of national regional disaster medical emergency, including the National Ministry of Health, Provincial Health Office, Army General Logistics Department of the Ministry of Health, Ministry of

Health, Joint Logistics Department of Military, and part of the rescue squad commander; (3) data on the national pumping group, local disaster emergency medical rescue forces, and the wounded admitted to the hospital; (4) interviews with medical experts and people in charge of emergency medical rescue workers at all levels; (5) forum for wounded individuals admitted to the hospital, rescue squad, and emergency medical personnel at all levels of command; (6) questionnaires for the medical support team, medical staff air transit station, local rescue workers, victims, and so on; and (7) related document reports.

1.2.4.3 Document Retrieval

We retrieved information from ProQuest, PubMed, and Chinese Biomedical Literature Database with the following search terms: Wenchuan earthquake or Yushu earthquake or earthquake and medical rescue or earthquake and management or earthquake and casualty or earthquake and evacuation or earthquake and public health or earthquake and PTSD or earthquake and health policy. These search terms produced a preliminary set of articles consistent with the study purpose. Then, we selected strong research from the preliminary articles that met content standards as references. Meanwhile, the research group searched other relevant information on hand, such as documents, statistics, announcements, special reports, news reports, evaluation reports, conference information, and publications issued by the China's State Council, the Chinese Ministry of Health, Government of Sichuan Province, the Qinghai provincial government, relief medical treatment groups, the earthquake rescue teams, and so on.

References

Gautschi, Oliver P et al. Earthquakes and trauma: review of triage and injury-specific, immediate care. Prehospital Disaster Med. 23.02(2008):195–201.

Kang P, Zhang L, Liang W, Zhu Z, Liu Y, Liu X, Yang H. Medical evacuation management and clinical characteristics of 3,255 inpatients after the 2010 Yushu earthquake in China. J Trauma Acute Care Surg. 2012;72(6):1626–33.

Zhang L, Liu Y, Liu X, Zhang Y. Rescue efforts management and characteristics of casualties of the Wenchuan earthquake in China. Emerg Med J: EMJ. 2011;28(7):618–22.

Zhang L, Liu X, Li Y, Liu Y, Liu Z, Lin J, Shen J, Tang X, Zhang Y, Liang W. Emergency medical rescue efforts after a major earthquake: lessons from the 2008 Wenchuan earthquake. Lancet. 2012;379(9818):853–61.

Chapter 2
Modeling the Occurrences of Earthquake Casualties

Zhipeng Liu and Lulu Zhang

Abstract In the short period after the earthquake, the outside relief forces know nothing about the casualties in the stricken area, which causes a lot of trouble to the medical relief work. Analyzing the impact factors of earthquake casualties, finding the earthquake casualties occurrence pattern, establishing the casualties model, and predicting the earthquake casualties have a significant impact on the rapid implementation of the earthquake medical relief and saving casualties.

After many factors of seismic casualties such as earthquake magnitude, building damage after the earthquake, earthquake occurrence time, personnel in the room rate, medical relief situation, and casualty evacuation situation were analyzed, we selected appropriate variables, using data of Yushu earthquake casualty, and established a Pareto model in MATLAB software. Through analyzing simulated earthquake casualty incidence, we expected earthquake casualty rescue efficiency can be improved to some extent.

2.1 Introduction

2.1.1 Background

2.1.1.1 Earthquakes and Consequent Casualties

Earthquakes are one of the most threatening natural disasters, as they are both sudden and unpredictable (Yi 2010). With devastating power, earthquakes can destroy buildings and infrastructure, resulting in casualties and economic loss. In addition to causing heavy casualties themselves, they are often accompanied by secondary disasters, such as fire damage, pollution, toxic and hazardous substances, mudslides, lake,

Z. Liu
Department of Military Health Service, College of Military Health Service, Second Military Medical University, Yangpu, Shanghai, China

L. Zhang (✉)
Department of Military Health Service, College of Military Health Service, Second Military Medical University, Shanghai, China
e-mail: zllrmit@aliyun.com

© Springer Science+Business Media Dordrecht 2016
L. Zhang (ed.), *Modeling the Injury Flow and Treatment after Major Earthquakes*, DOI 10.1007/978-94-017-7527-4_2

Table 2.1 The seven most deadly earthquakes since 2001 (EM-DAT)

Date	Country	Disaster type	Death rate (%)	Persons dead or missing	Affected persons	Economic loss (millions)
01/26/2001	India	Earthquake	0.32	20,005	6,321,812	2623
12/26/2003	Iran	Earthquake	10.01	26,796	267,628	500
12/26/2004	Indonesia	Earthquake with tsunami	31.10	165,708	532,898	4451.6
10/08/2005	Pakistan	Earthquake	1.43	73,338	5,128,309	5200
05/12/2008	China	Earthquake	0.19	87,476	45,976,596	85,000
01/12/2010	Haiti	Earthquake	6.02	222,570	3,700,000	8000
03/11/2011	Japan	Earthquake with tsunami	5.70	28,050	492,000	309,000

Table 2.2 Earthquake casualties in China between 2000 and 2010 (China Earthquake Networks Center)

Year	Number of earthquakes	Injured	Deaths
2000	10	2987	10
2001	12	750	9
2002	5	362	2
2003	21	7465	319
2004	11	696	8
2005	13	882	15
2006	10	229	25
2007	3	422	3
2008	17	374,176	69,197
2009	8	407	3
2010	12	13,795	2705

landslides, and plague, which lead to significant damage to residents' production and living areas. Coastal or deep-sea earthquakes may also cause tsunamis, leading to more casualties. Between 2001 and 2011, there have been 16 great earthquakes of more than 1000 deaths worldwide. The total death count was 700,000, and 70 million people were affected, with economic losses totaling $430 billion (Table 2.1).

China is located at the intersection of two seismic zones—the circum-Pacific seismic zone and the Eurasian seismic zone. It is severely affected by earthquakes, with high-frequency, high-intensity, widely distributed seismic intensity and superficial quake sources. Since the twentieth century, approximately 35 % of earthquakes greater than magnitude 7 on the Richter scale that have occurred worldwide have been in China. From 1949 to 1991, the total deaths from earthquakes accounted for 54 % of the total number of deaths from all kinds of natural disasters. Since 1949, there have been 59 earthquakes of at least 6.5 magnitude. The two largest, the Tangshan earthquake and the Wenchuan earthquake, resulted in 24.2 million and 6.9 million deaths, respectively, with as many as 164,000 and 374,000 injuries. From 2000 to 2010, China had more than 50 million casualties due to earthquakes, representing a serious threat to people's lives (Table 2.2).

2.1.1.2 Occurrence Patterns of Earthquake Casualties

After an earthquake suddenly occurs, most people are unable to leave buildings in sufficient time and are ultimately trapped or buried beneath. Some are quickly rescued by local rescuers, but a considerable number of people remain buried inside damaged buildings. Shortly after the earthquake, the outside rescue force has minimal understanding of the situation of the stricken area (e.g., disaster area, casualties, rescue force needs, and relief supply needs). Even after outside rescue forces run into the disaster areas, they still need a few hours to several days to clarify the situation. This directly affects the earthquake relief command layer, who has difficulty making rescue decisions. With mass casualties following the earthquake, the medical demand peaks in the first 24–48 h. In the 1988 Armenia earthquake, 97 % of the wounded were hospitalized in 6 days (Klain et al. 1990). Pretto's study (Pretto et al. 1994) showed that timely medical treatment within 6 h after earthquakes can save the lives of many wounded individuals. Therefore, timely and effective medical rescue of the wounded is critical. According to the available information, analysis of factors affecting seismic casualties, discovering the occurrence pattern of casualties, and establishing a casualty occurrence model can predict the distribution of the number and type of earthquake victims relatively accurately for quick implementation of earthquake medical rescue, guiding disaster relief personnel to save lives of the wounded. Therefore, establishing a strong predictive model to predict earthquake casualty changes has always been a hot research topic.

Factors affecting the occurrence of wounded individuals following an earthquake have long been studied internationally. The focal depth of the earthquake itself, the intensity, the local geological conditions, and so on will affect the number of wounded individuals, while local population density and age structure will also affect occurrence of casualties. In the 1990s, Schultz (1996) discovered that in earthquakes with substantial numbers of casualties, the number of wounded individuals concentrated within the first 24–48 h shows rapid growth and medical demand peaks in this period. From a survey investigating treatment of wounded individuals following the 2005 Pakistan earthquake (Mulvey et al. 2008), the number of wounded showed a clear linear growth pattern in the first 72 h after the earthquake. After observing medical treatment following several earthquakes, the international community has generally concluded that the occurrence pattern of wounded earthquake victims shows stepwise variation. Studies on the distribution of casualty locations have come to the following conclusions: (1) It is a priority to figure out the earthquake situation and the local geological conditions. (2) After the earthquake, most of the wounded are concentrated in the vicinity of collapsed buildings, but not evenly distributed in the affected area. (3) The ability to quickly clear the position of collapsed buildings can effectively reduce the waiting time for treatment. (4) The early establishment of geographic information systems (GISs) can play a role in disaster relief. (5) David Alexander (2000) of the University of Massachusetts pointed out that the basic types of geographical distribution of earthquake injuries are in line with the Gaussian distribution, binomial distribution, exponential distribution, and so on.

After the Wenchuan earthquake, scholars who investigated local buildings and the occurrence of wounded individuals concluded that construction materials and traumatic brain injury occurrence were correlated. In our group's investigation, the hardest hit province following the Wenchuan earthquake was Sichuan, where the casualties were greatest in Wenchuan, Mianzhu, Beichuan, Shifang, Guangyuan, Green River, Chengdu, Mao County, and Dujiangyan regions, accounting for 77.10 % of the total deaths (He et al. 2008). Because the earthquake struck in the afternoon, the casualties occurred in densely populated areas such as schools and hospitals. The students of Sichuan province accounted for 7 % of total deaths, and persons above 75 and between 10 and 14 years accounted for a large proportion of the wounded. Within 2 weeks after the earthquake, the reported number of casualties continued to grow, reaching a peak 2 weeks later (May 26).

The impact factors of earthquake casualties gradually improved, and the dynamic varying pattern of the occurrence of wounded individuals also gets people's further attention. It becomes increasingly necessary to combine the two sides effectively to more accurately predict casualties before earthquakes and guide rescuers' earthquake emergency relief to save more lives.

2.1.2 Current Situation and Literature Review

2.1.2.1 Dynamic Pattern of Earthquake Casualties Varies with Time

Why Earthquake Casualty Patterns Are Dynamic

At the moment an earthquake strikes, a large number of deaths instantly occur and many people are buried in collapsed buildings. Before being rescued and transferred to a safe and stable health-care environment, the lives of buried persons are in a gradually deteriorating state. For some seriously injured individuals, if treatment is not received in a timely matter, their wounds may be quickly aggravated and become fatal. In the Tangshan earthquake, the survival rate of the wounded dug out within the first half hour after the earthquake was almost 100 %. However, 6 h later, this rate was reduced to less than 10 %. The quickly organized self-help and mutual aid of local people after the earthquake and rapid treatment of external earthquake rescue teams could save those seriously injured in the effective treatment period to avoid unnecessary deaths. These factors contribute to the dynamic variation in earthquake casualty occurrence, thereby forming patterns.

The Dynamic Pattern of Earthquake Casualty Occurrence

Generally speaking, earthquake casualties rise as rescue forces continuously come into the disaster area. The casualty pattern is clearly divided into a "rapid growth period" and a "sustained period" by an obvious inflection point in time. The time growth inflection point is related with the rescue force covering speed and earthquake situation. The period before the inflection point is the high-speed "growth period," and after the inflection point is the "sustained period" for casualties. The casualty growth inflection point is related with seismic scales: The greater the scale of the earthquake, the more casualties there are and the later the inflection point comes out. Conversely, a small-scale earthquake has a smaller number of casualties and the inflection point occurs earlier.

The occurrence of earthquake casualties is affected by numerous factors. These factors include the earthquake situation, the local environment, the population structure, and the rescue behavior, among other factors. Running a systematic analysis of these factors would contribute to anti-seismic and quakeproof work and provide parameters for models predicting casualties.

2.1.2.2 Factors Affecting Earthquake Casualty Occurrence

The Earthquake Situation

The Seismic Scale

M is the scale of the earthquake, short for earthquake magnitude; it is based on the energy released by each seismic activity, measured with the seismometer. The larger the earthquake is, the larger the magnitude figure shows. With a magnitude increase of 1, the energy released by an earthquake increased by 32 times. Because it has no direct link with the physical characteristics of the source, the moment magnitude (M_w) scale is more often used now.

Earthquake magnitude itself is an important parameter indicating destructive energy, which greatly influences earthquake casualties. By analyzing 100 years of major global seismic situations between 1890 and 1989 (Oike 1991), it was found that the smaller magnitude earthquakes ($M \leq 4$) generally do not cause death, while in larger magnitude earthquakes ($M > 4$), the number of deaths grew with increases in earthquake magnitude, with even minor changes causing tenfold increases in the number of deaths. With different times or different locations, earthquakes of the same scale cause substantial differences in death toll and there is no clear linear relationship between earthquake magnitude and death number. Further, with earthquake magnitudes between 4 and 8, the death toll level was 10^1, 10^2, 10^3, 10^4, and 10^5, respectively, indicating the maximum number of deaths increases with earthquake magnitude.

Seismic Intensity

Seismic intensity refers to the damage intensity to the surface area and a variety of buildings following an earthquake. After an earthquake occurs, the seismic intensity of areas with different distances to epicenters could be assessed according to changes of the surface and the degree of building damage. The isoseismal lines could be drawn to describe the extent of the damage. Thus, the seismic intensity is mainly used for explaining the impact of the earthquake. The seismic intensity of a region is related not only with the energy released from the earthquake, the distance from the epicenter, and the focal depth but also with geological conditions of pathways in which the seismic wave is propagated and characteristics of buildings.

1. Comparing across different population densities

By dividing regions in advance by population density as (1) city; (2) township (population density $\geq 100/km^2$); and (3) rural (population density <100 people/km^2), Zou Qijia (1990) analyzed seismic intensity and casualties in Chinese major earthquakes between 1966 and 1976. It was clearly found that with the same population density, the casualty rate changes with intensity, showing a significant positive correlation.

2. Comparing across different building structures

The anti-seismic capacity of the building structure has a substantial impact on casualties. Coburn (Coburn 1989) summarized the mortality rates with different housing structures in several earthquakes in the 1980s. After excluding the impact of anti-seismic capacities of building structures, with increased earthquake intensity, mortality rates showed an increasing trend with a clear correlation.

Timing of Earthquakes

Earthquake occurrence time also has a significant impact on casualties. Coburn found that timing has a clear impact on the number of earthquake casualties by analyzing the occurrence times and death toll of earthquakes in Japan, Turkey, Greece, and so on. Casualties caused by earthquakes around midnight will be higher than at other times, even more than double, especially in comparison to midday. Okada (1992) indicated that the impact of timing on casualties can be accounted for by two main factors. First, timing determines the number of people indoors. The rate of people in residences is highest at midnight, and thus, if an earthquake occurs at this time, it can easily cause massive casualties. Second, if the earthquake occurs at night, people are often in a state of deep sleep and their mobility is lowest. When the earthquake occurs, it is often difficult to find shelter in a timely matter, thereby increasing casualties.

Environments of Stricken Areas

Geographical Environment

After the earthquake, fires often occur. This may be because stricken areas have large amounts of combustible materials, such as chemical plants, timber mills, and so on. If the earthquake occurs during dry, hot, and windy weather, and the local extinguishing capacities are poor, the road damage is serious, the traffic is standstill, and rescue forces are unable to quickly reach the affected area, the occurrence of large fires in stricken areas becomes probable. The most typical example is the 8.3-magnitude earthquake that occurred in Japan's Kanto region on September 1, 1923 (Dezhi 1990). The earthquake occurred at noon, and people mainly used flames to cook. After the earthquake, the flames got out of control, burning many houses. Among all deaths, 95 % were burned or suffocated or drowned to avoid the fire.

Earthquakes occurring in the coastal areas often cause oceanic plates to move, submarine faulting, and terrain moves up or down steeply, causing a huge tsunami that inundates stricken areas, leading to even more casualties than caused by the earthquake itself. For example, an M9 earthquake occurred undersea near the island of Sumatra on December 26, 2004, causing a huge tsunami that swept across Southeast Asia, south of the Indian Ocean, and far beyond the scope of the earthquake, killing nearly 300,000. It was concluded that the larger the tsunami, the more deaths there are by analyzing the deaths caused by earthquakes and tsunamis in Japan.

Due to the special geographical environment, other secondary disasters caused by the earthquake, such as landslides, avalanche lakes, and so on, would cause tremendous threat to life to earthquake survivors and rescue workers if not promptly resolved, often causing more casualties again, exacerbating the situation. For example, in 1933 (Gongxu 1983), the occurrence of the Sichuan Diexi M7.5 earthquake caused mountain collapse and formed four avalanche lakes. Then, the dams burst and a flood was formed, drowning more than 2500 people, which accounted for 40 % of all deaths.

Building Structure and Rate of Collapse

A large proportion of earthquake casualties are not caused by the earthquake movement itself but by the collapsing houses caused by earthquakes. For example, the Taiwan ChiChi earthquake (Zhi 2006) caused 2492 deaths, and 94 % of deaths were attributed to building collapse, of which adobe houses accounted for 41 %, brick (including strengthening of masonry) houses accounted for 15 %, and reinforced concrete buildings accounted for 17 %. After the 2008 Wenchuan earthquake, the deaths related with buildings collapsing in Jiangyou, An County, and Qingchuan and most other accounted for up to or more than 70 % of all deaths (Wang et al. 2009). With the earthquake magnitude and seismic intensity fixed, the anti-seismic capacity of the buildings played a decisive role on rates of houses collapsing. The destruction rate of buildings without seismic protection was 10.88 % (Baitao and Guixin 2010), much higher than that for buildings with reinforcement, causing a large number of casualties. Shiono summarized the relationships between mortality rates (fatality rate, FR) and the collapse rate of 11 types of buildings (collapsed rate, CR): $FR = FR_{100} * (CR/100)^n$ (Shiono et al. 1991). FR_{100} is the mortality rate when the collapse rate is 100 %, which is mainly determined by the anti-seismic capacities of building structures; n refers to an index that relies on different types of building construction.

When completely collapsed, gravel and brick houses had the highest mortality rates, reaching 30 % and 25 %, respectively. This may be because, in the case of complete collapse, gravel and brick houses have smaller debris, leading to greater damage, and the lack of walls to form a protective structure leads to people being completely buried after collapse. Living space is small, space is limited, and oxygen is lacking, and uncovering the buried is extremely difficult.

Demographic Structure of Stricken Areas

Population Density and Structure

The impact of population density on the number of seismic casualties is clear. With the same intensity, the higher the population density, the more casualties will occur. Thus, urban casualties > town casualties > rural casualties. Further, when earthquakes strike areas with higher indoor population density, collapsed buildings affect more population, producing a higher casualty rate.

Beyond the effect of population density, population age and gender also influence casualties. In general, due to male physique generally stronger than that of females, escape is easier and chance of survival after injury is greater, thereby leading to a higher rate of casualties in females. Also, due to the weaker physique of children and elderly individuals, these populations are more likely to get hurt and have a poorer prognosis (Zhang et al. 2012).

Population Education

Yokoyama (1992) simulated and analyzed the evacuation route and time in the earthquake by using maze experiments. It was discovered that the number of evacuating people was approximately normally distributed with evacuation time and the maximum came out between 100 and 250 s. However, the earthquake ground shaking time is generally in the tens of seconds and only a small number of people could run out of the buildings safely.

Running out of the building in a hurry when the quake struck is often the incorrect decision. When the earthquake happened, many people wasted these precious tens of seconds running out into the road and lost hope of survival in the process. The lack of proper rational understanding of earthquakes often results in excessive panic, leading to unnecessary casualties. Therefore, in areas where earthquakes are common, launching anti-seismic education can help to establish proper seismic psychology to avoid people taking irrational escape measures and can largely reduce earthquake casualties.

Medical Relief Work

Echelon Treatment After Earthquakes (Yanling 2010)

1. Theory of echelon treatment

In mass casualty events such as earthquakes, local medical resources work overtime and still cannot meet all the needs of the wounded and it is thus necessary that some of these injuries will be transferred to other medical institutions. The "echelon treatment" principle holds that for wounded treatment, a phased evacuation is a continuous process and should take the form of a stepped approach, and the amount of assistance requiring surgery will differ all stages of medical evacuation and across casualty evacuation methods. Following reasonable distribution of wounded individuals, effective use of limited medical resources early in disasters, such as earthquakes, can stabilize the wounded after injury, effectively reducing casualties.

Disaster medical rescue will be divided into a two- or three-level hierarchical treatment. For major disasters, it can be divided into three treatment level: The first treatment level is emergency treatment, the second is early-stage treatment, and the third is specialist treatment. Due to the insufficiency of medical resource in the earthquake-stricken areas, the first-level and secondary-level treatments are mainly launched in the affected areas.

Self-help of the wounded, as well as mutual aid organizations and aid forces, provide first aid. Emergency treatment including on-site treatment (bleeding, bandaging, fixed, etc.), triage, anti-infective, anti-shock, the implementation of emergency lifesaving surgery, and a 1-week stay governance can cure those who have been lightly wounded. Usually by forces responsible for organizing grassroots medical service institutions, local grassroots rural hospitals will assist. The basic treatment principle is to keep more people live. Before transporting the wounded people to hospitals, the trauma and crisis situation, such as shock and suffocation, must be seriously treated with these emergency treatment measures. If there is no pre-fast, efficient hospital care, individuals may die at the site of the wound occurrence or in transit, and even with advanced hospital equipment, technology wise, it is difficult to revive in such circumstances. Therefore, early treatment of the wounded is one of the most important factors.

The influences of hospitals and disaster medical station in the affected areas on the triage and early treatment of wounded are crucial. There exists a range of specialist treatment, including emergency specialist treatment and improved specialist treatment, and the former principle of early treatment refers to the implementation of various specialties, such as debridement, anti-shock, amputation, and damage control surgery. Either by the military field medical teams or by various specialty surgical teams responsible for implementation, these treatments can also be carried out by the local hospital in more than two units. Improvement mainly refers to specialist treatment after definitive surgery and carrying out a variety of injury prevention measures. Further, timely comprehensive anti-shock and anti-infection treatment by local tertiary hospitals, specialist hospitals, and military hospitals is performed.

2. Triage methods

International earthquake disaster relief mainly used the Simple Triage and Rapid Treatment (START triage) method, especially in Europe and North America. Disaster triage methods used in the earthquake scene are enacted in accordance with START. For earthquakes in Armenia, the wounded are divided by the emergency medical personnel into treatment, delayed treatment, and expectant treatment categories. European and American countries have established START, JumpSTART, secondary assessment of victim endpoint (SAVE), triage sieve, and the Sacco triage method as common triage criteria (Yehezkel et al. 2006; Hamilton et al. 2009; On-Line CEU; Romig; Hodgetts and Mackway-Jones 1995; Jenkins et al. 2008; Garner et al. 2001).

3. Future trend of echelon treatment

Since the 1990s, due to the proposed development of air transport technology and research, medical air transport issues and solutions and air evacuation to the earthquake relief in several foreign countries will further simplify the classification into a two-level treatment evacuation ladder, that is, rescuing and fast specialist treatment, which greatly improves the prognosis for wounded individuals, especially those who have been critically wounded. The general view is that under adequate conditions, a two treatment level system could be employed with rapid evacuation transport (early treatment ladder omitted).

Medical Treatment in Stricken Areas

If rescue workers arrive to the scene in time, a large number of wounded individuals buried after the earthquake can be treated appropriately in hospitals. It is noteworthy that due to the hysteresis of the external disaster relief forces' arrival, the self-help and mutual help of survivors in the earthquake area played an important role. According to rough estimates, in the Soviet earthquake, people's behavior and mutual aid treatment accounted for 95 % of all rescued (Hongfu et al. 2011).

Medical Treatment in Rear Hospitals Receiving the Injured

For most of the wounded, after positive first aid following the earthquake and attainment of stable vital signs, the issue becomes the recovery of maximum possible damaged functionality. A small part of the critically wounded require complex rescue and major support from medical equipment in rear hospitals to have a chance at survival. Thus, in rear hospitals, when receiving the wounded, there is a need for treatment, including postoperative rehabilitation training and psychological counseling, as well as hospital infection control during treatment, in order to save lives. The main purpose here is to reduce mortality and disability of the wounded and improve the quality of the rehabilitation of the wounded.

As most wounded individuals in earthquakes experience trauma and crush injuries, surgery is one of the main measures involved in hospitals following earthquakes. Further, because the wounded experience complex injuries, wounds, and are exposed to pollution, infection is often accompanied by complex and rare bacteria that are resistant to nosocomial infection control. To a large extent, this determines the posttreatment effects. After crush injury, victims can experience crush injury syndrome, which is caused by renal failure, which often overshadows trauma and illness. If this is not detected and treated in a timely matter, it will seize the wounded, leaving them with just a few hours to live. The rehabilitation of the wounded past the critical stage is an essential step in disaster relief. Further, emergency treatment and prevention of infectious diseases, as well as concern about the survival rate of early complications compared with the purpose of rehabilitation, is to obtain short- and long-term functional optimization.

Other Factors

Whether there is prewarning before an earthquake can also influence seismic casualties. For example, before the Liaoning HaiCheng 7.3 earthquake in February 4, 1975, the local earthquake department accurately predicted the occurrence of the earthquake and the government decisively evacuated all residents, greatly reducing casualties, as only 1328 people died. If there was no timely evacuation of local residents, the HaiCheng earthquake would have likely caused 1.3 million deaths.

2.1.3 Objective and Significance

2.1.3.1 Objective

Earthquake casualties are at the forefront of earthquake emergency medical rescue, and they are also a key element of the success of the earthquake relief operations. Compared with other earthquake-prone countries, the study of the occurrence of natural disasters with regard to medical rescue of the wounded is still in its infancy in China. Objective and accurate simulation models to predict the occurrence of earthquake victims have not yet been established, and China remains focused on the study of descriptive statistics of the sick and wounded. Due to policy, human, material, and other factors, it is difficult to study earthquake casualties on account of the lack of large-scale multicenter comprehensive surveys at the national level. Thus, injury characteristics and laws of the occurrence of wounded individuals in earthquakes cannot be analyzed as a whole. Our previous theoretical review demonstrates "two phases" of changes in casualties, which was verified by the trend of domestic earthquake casualty analysis. These "two" laws were assessed in a systematic review, and the advantages and disadvantages of existing prediction methods were analyzed and summarized. We conducted a retrospective analysis of field research of the Yushu earthquake to investigate the basic characteristics of the distribution of earthquake victims in time, space, and the proportion of wounded casualties. We also investigated the composition of Ministry injury class types and other characteristics, and the study concluded the previous earthquake casualty prediction model by establishing a comprehensive predictive model of dynamic earthquake casualty rescue behavior. Timely guidance of the work of rescue forces will provide a scientific basis for predicting the occurrence of the wounded and rational allocation of health resources.

2.1.3.2 Significance

In our previous study, based on the application of mathematical modeling techniques and methods, systems evaluation, and qualitative research, we used descriptive analysis and correlation analysis to compare domestic and foreign earthquake casualty trends, in-depth analysis of seismic verification of casualties, and the "two-phase" law. The review summarized factors affecting casualties in the Yushu earthquake based on empirical analysis and the strengths and weaknesses of past earthquake casualty prediction models and derived a prediction method for casualty occurrence using a Pareto-simulated dynamic model in order to provide an objective basis for scientific rescue work.

2.2 Data Resource Used in the Model

2.2.1 Utilization of the Current Data Resource

1. The data and materials of the basic information on the injured and their medical treatment from all previous major earthquakes worldwide, including data like "The earthquake case of China" from a retrieval of information on the Internet
2. More than 100 copies of documents, reports, and statistics on emergency medical rescue, basic disease information of the sick and injured, and treatment conditions and other earthquake relief information on the Yushu earthquake from the Ministry of Health of the People's Republic of China
3. More than 50 copies of the related public documents on the emergency medical rescue of Wenchuan, participation in the Yushu earthquake relief by the People's Liberation Army of China, and more than 80 copies of earthquake relief brief reports from Chinese military medical universities
4. Studies on the occurrence of casualties and their patterns from Chinese earthquake emergency medical rescue books (e.g., "the medical support of Military Operations Other Than War") that have been openly published in the last 20 years.

2.2.2 Data Source from Field Surveys

As a part of Yushu earthquake relief emergency medical rescue field investigation, the field investigation on the sick and injured following the Yushu earthquake is divided into three stages.

2.2.2.1 Investigation Time and Objects

First, in October 2010, the research group went to the Ministry of Health of China (Beijing) for Yushu earthquake emergency medical rescue data collection and assessment for 5 days. Data related to the sick and injured and basic information about treatment included the following: first, the related documents released by the Ministry of Health of China; second, the duty log on the Yushu earthquake relief from the Ministry of Health of China; third, the reported information statistical tables of the Ministry of Health of China; and fourth, all the meeting summaries of the Qinghai Yushu earthquake health emergency leading group.

Second, in December 2010, the research group went to Xining Qinghai Province and conducted one week of retrospective field research. The research subjects were primarily medical relief agencies, health administration agencies, and medical and rescue personnel. The research group investigated the Emergency Management Office and the Bureau of Medical Affairs of the Qinghai Province Health Department, the Health Bureau of the Yushu Autonomous Prefecture (during the investigation, the relevant personnel were training in Xining, Qinghai Province), and other health administration agencies. The research group also investigated the medical and health institutions that supported the stricken area of Yushu in Qinghai Province, which included more than 10 units, such as the Qinghai Provincial People's Hospital, the affiliated hospital of Qinghai University, Qinghai Red Cross Hospital, People's Armed Police Corps Hospital of Qinghai Province, and the Qinghai Province Center for Disease Control and Prevention.

Finally, in January and February 2011, the research group conducted an additional investigation in Sichuan, Shaanxi, Gansu, and Tibet Autonomous Region to conduct supplementary research in these four provinces. The research subjects were primarily hospitals that admitted sick and injured individuals who were evacuated from Yushu.

2.2.2.2 Survey Methodology

The survey mainly used expert interviews, small meetings, questionnaire surveys, and other forms. The subjects of the expert interviews were primarily leaders of the Qinghai Provincial Health Department and Yushu Prefecture Health Bureau, in three separate interviews. The subjects of the small discussion meetings included a total of more than 40 health officers, medical personnel, and health supervisors in Yushu earthquake relief, which were also conducted three times. The contents of all the interviews were recorded in text and audio, which were organized at the end of the study. Those participating in the questionnaire surveys were mainly earthquake emergency medical rescue medical personnel, including more than 300 medical staff in Qinghai Province and more than 120 Yushu county medical staff. Phone and Internet questionnaires were the main methods of conducting supplementary research. These were commissioned by the Health Departments in Sichuan, Shaanxi, Gansu, and Tibet, who distributed and collected the questionnaires and then returned them to the research group by email or mail.

2.2.2.3 Survey Contents

First, surveys investigated the occurrence of injury in the earthquake-stricken areas. Second, they investigated the nationwide deployment situation of China, the local disaster emergency medical and relief forces of the stricken areas, and the rear hospital that treated the sick and injured who had been evacuated from stricken areas. Third, interviews were conducted with more than 60 medical experts and emergency medical rescue work personnel at all levels. Fourth, more than 10 symposia were conducted with the hospitals that admitted the wounded; these included medical relief commanding personnel of rescue teams and other medical relief agencies at all levels. Fifth, we examined more than 500 copies of relevant statements and reports.

2.2.2.4 Quality Control

In the interviews and surveys, we conducted detailed data collection and detailed interview outlines, discussed the issues one by one in accordance with the outlines, and listened to the views and opinions of the interviewees and conference staff. We then recorded and organized the data. Before conducting questionnaire surveys, the significance of the survey research should be explained in detail, and the key topics were explained one by one to ensure that the subjects filled out the questionnaires appropriately. During the questionnaire surveys with the local medical staff of Yushu county, work staff from the local health bureau helped the research group explain the questionnaire item by item to avoid language-related problems.

2.2.3 Collection of Literature

The key words "seismic (earthquake), injuries (casualty), impact factors (affecting factor), modeling (modeling), and forecasting (predicting)" were used to retrieve and view articles from Medline, ProQuest, PubMed, and Chongqing VIP periodical database, Chinese Biomedical Literature Database, and so on from 1970 to 2012. Then, more than 60 studies were screened out because they focused on factors affecting seismic casualties and modeling and simulation of the occurrence of earthquake casualties worldwide.

2.3 Modeling the Occurrence of Earthquake Casualties in MATLAB

2.3.1 Selection of Variables

According to the literature review and analysis of factors affecting earthquake casualties, the research group selected earthquake magnitude, degree of damage to buildings, number of people indoors, earthquake time, medical relief staff's rescue situations, and evacuation of casualties as covariates along with time after the earthquake in accordance with their importance in determining the occurrence of earthquake casualties. These covariates were entered into the hypothetical model to predict dynamic variation in earthquake casualties.

2.3.2 *Constructing the Model of Earthquake Casualty Occurrence*

2.3.2.1 Index and State Function of Earthquake Casualties

Earthquake Casualties Index

To effectively analyze and express the state of earthquake casualties, the research group introduced a casualties index from elsewhere, denoted by C (casualty), on behalf of the degree to which persons buried beneath buildings after the earthquake were injured (Zhao et al. 1998). $C=0$ means no injuries and $C=1$ means that the person is dead (Table 2.3).

Earthquake Casualties State Function

Casualties state function:

$$C(t)=\left(C_0^{1/n}+S_i t\right)^n$$

C_0 is the initial casualty index, $C_0 \in [0,1]$, S_i is the environmental parameter when the stranded environment classification value is i. n is a physical index, and depending on whether physical condition is good or bad, n can take 1.0, 1.5, 2.0, 2.5, or 3.0. t represents the time a person has been trapped.

2.3.2.2 The "Two-Phase" Pattern of Casualty Growth, Arrival Numbers of Medical Relief Staff, and Evacuation of the Injured

Through the analysis of the Yushu earthquake medical relief, it can be seen that the growth of casualties, the relief personnel arriving at the disaster area, and the injured who were evacuated by air presented a "two-phase" pattern, which is in line with the Pareto distribution.

Table 2.3 Earthquake casualties index

C I	0–0.1	0.1–0.3	0.3–0.6	0.6–0.9	0.9–1.0
Status	Not injured	Slightly injured	Moderately injured	Severely injured	Fatally injured

In the Pareto distribution, if X is a random variable, the probability distribution of X is as follows:

$$P(X > x) = \left(\frac{x}{x_{\min}}\right)^{-k},$$

$$p(x) = \begin{cases} 0, & if\, x < x_{\min}; \\ \frac{k x^{k}_{\min}}{x^{k+1}}, & if\, x > x_{\min}. \end{cases}$$

X is any number greater than X_{min}, and X_{min} is the smallest possible value of X (positive number). k is a positive parameter. The Pareto distribution curve family is parameterized by two quantities: X_{min} and k. The density distribution is the Pareto distribution, which is a continuous probability distribution. The "J_i Pufu Law," also known as the "zeta distribution," is also considered a Pareto distribution of the discrete probability distribution. A random variable to comply with the Pareto distribution has the expected value of $\frac{x_{\min} k}{k-1}$ (if $k \le 1$, the expected value is infinite) and the standard deviation of the random variable is $\frac{x_{\min}}{k-1}\sqrt{\frac{k}{k-2}}$ (if $k \le 1$, the standard deviation does not exist).

The probability density function of the Pareto distribution and the cumulative distribution function $\frac{k x_{\mathrm{m}}^{k}}{x^{k+1}} 1-\left(\frac{x_{\mathrm{m}}}{x}\right)^{k}$ were $\left(x \in [x_m; +\infty]\right)$.

2.3.2.3 Building the Dynamic Model

Considering the time at which the earthquake occurred, its intensity, and building destruction rate (there are different housing structures and anti-seismic capacity is different, so the damage rate will be different).

Daytime:

$$P_{\text{dead}} = \alpha e^{0.5(\sigma-7)} P_{\text{dest}}$$
$$P_{\text{inj}} = \beta e^{0.5(\sigma-7)} P_{\text{dest}}$$

Nighttime:

$$P_{\text{dead}} = \alpha \frac{\sigma - 4.76}{\sigma + 0.25} e^{0.75(\sigma-7)} P_{\text{des}}$$
$$P_{\text{inj}} = \frac{0.0686}{\sigma + 0.25} e^{0.75(\sigma-7)} P_{\text{des}}$$

When the earthquake occurred, the earthquake killed some people directly. The medical treatment was carried out on the injured and sick who were still alive. Further, each person's initial injured status and time trapped were different. The model assumes that the opportunity for every person to be searched out was the same and the probability of the medical relief team arriving is $p(t)$, which is a time-varying variable (with a longer time comes a greater probability of arrival). Therefore, whether the person could get treatment depends on their injured status, time trapped, and the time of arrival of the treatment teams. It is generally believed that if more than 7 days go by without being recovered, the injured can be considered dead, $P_{\text{live}}=0$.

$$P_{\text{live}} = P\left(y=t/x=t\right)C\left(t\right)$$

The number of persons being saved

$$S_{\text{live}} = P_{\text{live}} M_{\text{quake}} \left(1-P_{\text{inj}}\right)$$

is a random function that changes with time.

Then, the above functions were programmed in MATLAB to complete the construction of the model.

2.4 Simulation and Prediction of the Model

2.4.1 Simulation

After the program was set, the Yushu earthquake casualty occurrence was dynamically simulated, and the simulation results were obtained (Fig. 2.1).

As can be seen, the total number of people injured in the Yushu earthquake was 17,295, the total number of deaths was 4186, the number of the slightly injured persons was 7648, the number of moderately injured persons was 6741, the number of severely injured persons was 1802, and finally, the number enduring deadly injuries was 1104. The inflection point between the rapid growth period and the stable period of the injured saved was the sixth day after the earthquake. The actual number of injuries was 12,135, the number of deaths was 2968, and the number of individuals severely injured was 1434. The inflection point for the growth of the injured was also the sixth day after the earthquake.

It can be seen in the simulation of the model and the actual situation of the Yushu earthquake that the same order of magnitude was observed for the number of people injured, severely injured, and the number of deaths. The deviation was 42.52 % for the injured, 41.04 % for the deceased, and 23.01 % for the severely injured. The primary reasons may have been as follows: First, the model itself needs further adjustment; second, after the earthquake, the stricken area was in chaos and data

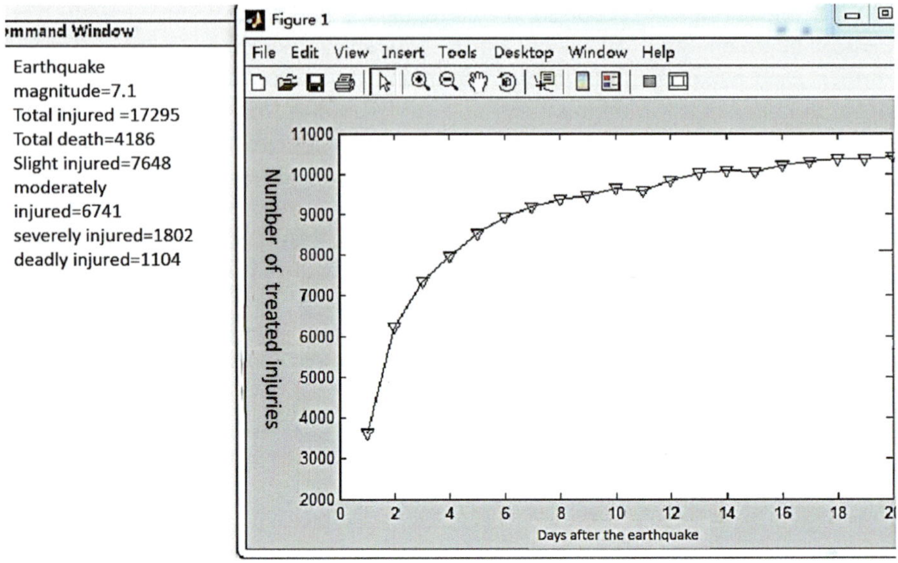

Fig. 2.1 The result of the model simulating the Yushu earthquake

collection did not correspond with the actual situation—the deviation may have occurred when constructing the model with inaccurate data; and third, the impact of the medical relief staff in the modeling might be derived from the delay caused by casualty evacuation.

2.4.2 *Predicting*

Based on the Yushu earthquake data, we thoroughly changed the relevant influencing factors in the model, and the evolution pattern of previous findings was simulated and verified.

2.4.2.1 Simulation and Prediction of Different Earthquake Magnitudes

The model that made predictions under different magnitudes could be obtained by changing the magnitude factors (Figs. 2.2, 2.3, 2.4, and 2.5).

As can be seen, with the different earthquake magnitudes, the overall numbers of casualties differ considerably. For example, with a magnitude of 5, only 1299 people were injured and 1427 people were killed (Fig. 2.2). With magnitude 9, 132,949 people were injured and 103,537 were killed. The population of Yushu autonomous prefecture was just 283,100, of which the total number of casualties resulting from a magnitude 9 earthquake would account for more than 80 % (Fig. 2.5).

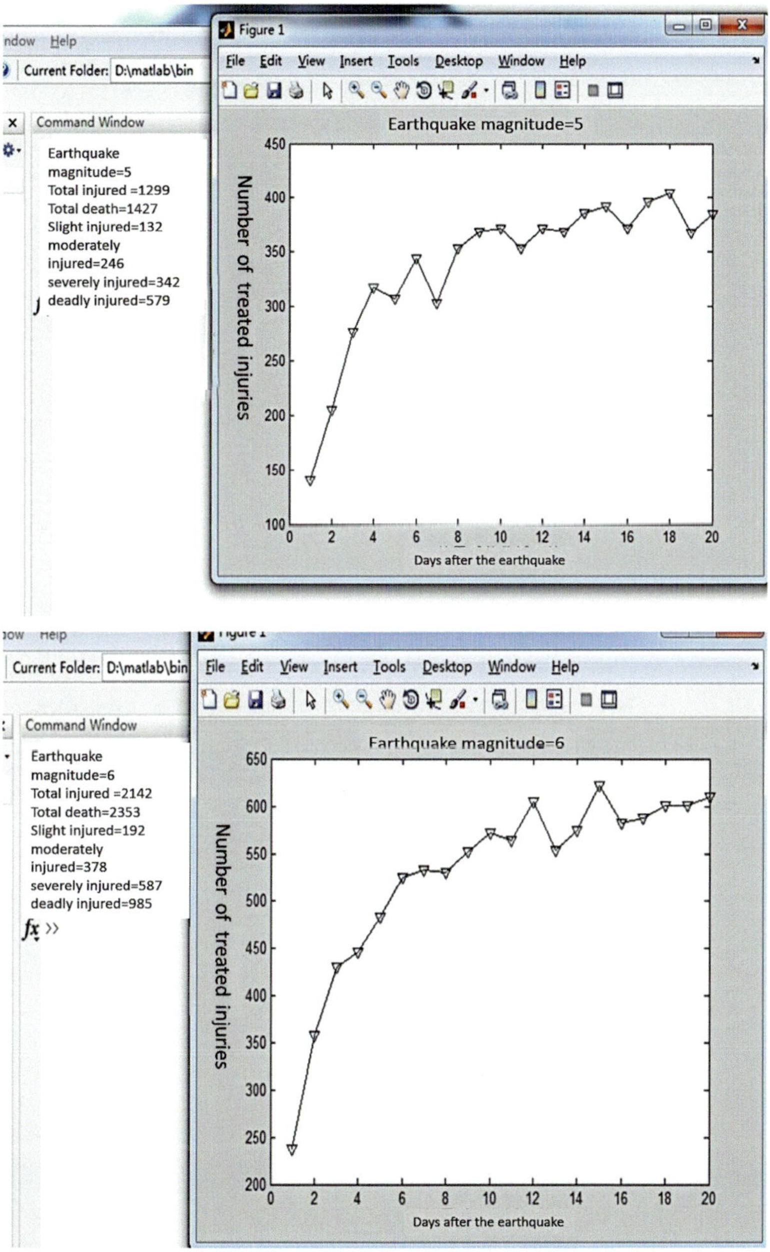

Fig. 2.2–2.5 Prediction results of the model with different earthquake magnitudes

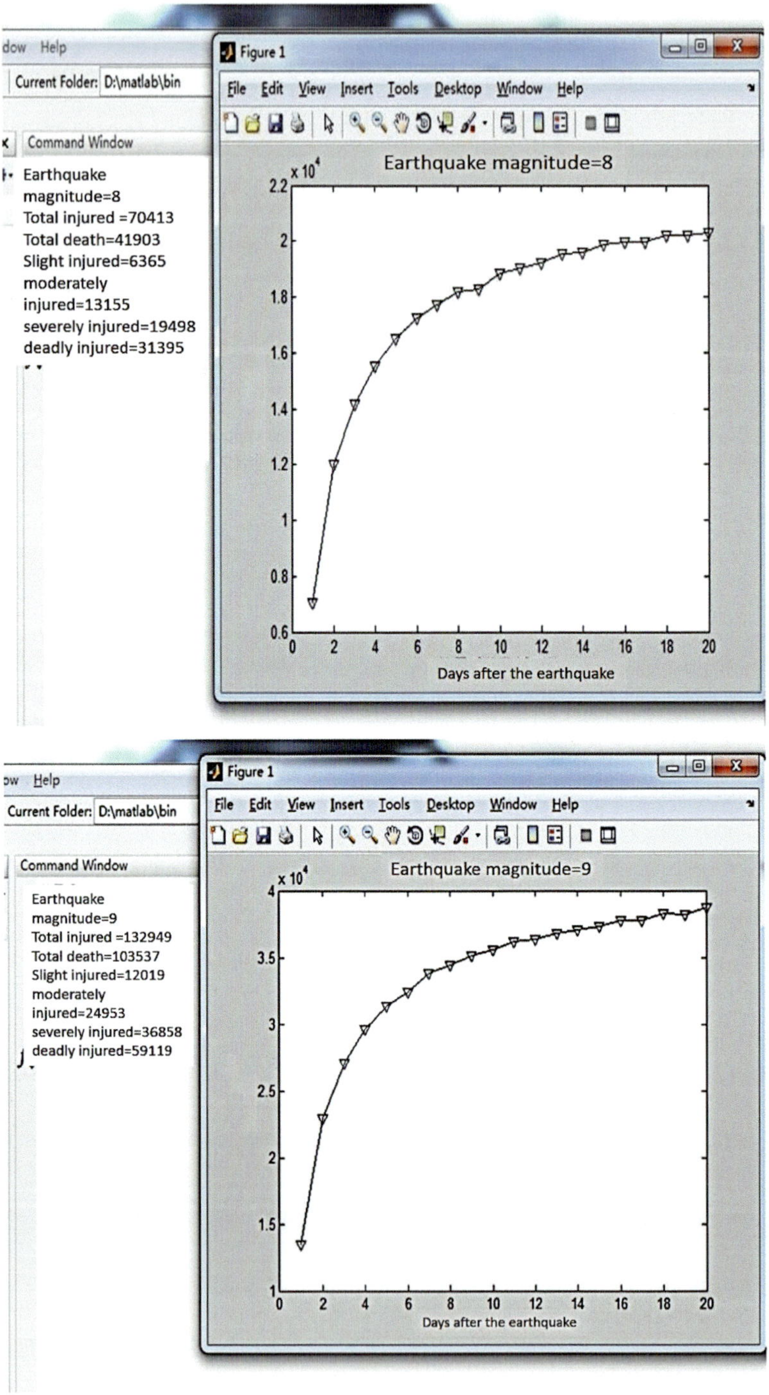

Fig. 2.2–2.5 (continued)

The rate at which the injured were saved daily was in line with the "two-phase" dynamic pattern. When the earthquake magnitude was 5, the inflection point was the fourth day after the earthquake, and the first 4 days constituted the rapid growth period for casualties (Fig. 2.2). The stable period began after the fourth day. When the magnitude was 6, the inflection point was the seventh day after the earthquake (Fig. 2.3), and for large-scale earthquakes (magnitude 8 or 9), the inflection point appeared later (both appearing on the eighth day in the prediction), and the curve is relatively smooth, with a long period of rapid growth and a less-obvious inflection point between the rapid growth period and the stable growth period (Figs. 2.4 and 2.5).

2.4.2.2 Simulation and Prediction with Different Arrival Speeds of Outside Support Forces

The impact of the arrival speed of medical relief staff on earthquake casualties has always been a hot research topic. The arrival speed of the medical relief staff was divided into three levels: all arrived within zero days (meaning that the local disaster medical relief force was able to meet the relief demand), all arrived within 1 day, and all arrived within 3 days. The model was then run again to simulate different arrival speeds of outside support forces.

The analysis of the simulation results demonstrates that if all the outside support forces arrive in the first 3 days after the earthquake, there is a significant impact on the medical treatment of the injured (Figs. 2.6, 2.7, and 2.8). Specifically, if the outside support medical forces arrive within the first 3 days, the total number of injured was just over 3700 and the death toll was more than 4000, only 52 % of the actual casualties, which is much better than the actual situation. Within the first 3 days of medical relief, if the outside medical personnel arrive later, the injury situation will deteriorate more quickly, and an increasingly number of people will die. After the fifth day following the earthquake, the arrival of the outside medical personnel could not prevent the deterioration of the injury and death. The highest number of deadly injuries was 1693, which occurred when the outside medical personnel arrived within 1 day (Fig. 2.6). This is likely because many individuals with severe injuries who might otherwise die could be saved if medical rescue arrive within 5–8 h after the earthquake. In other situations, a substantial number of dying individuals would have already died, thereby reducing the number of severe injuries.

It is evident that if the local disaster medical force can meet the basic medical needs of the injured, casualties and the severity of the injured can be greatly reduced. If all outside support forces arrive in the first 3 days after the earthquake, the number of injuries can be reduced.

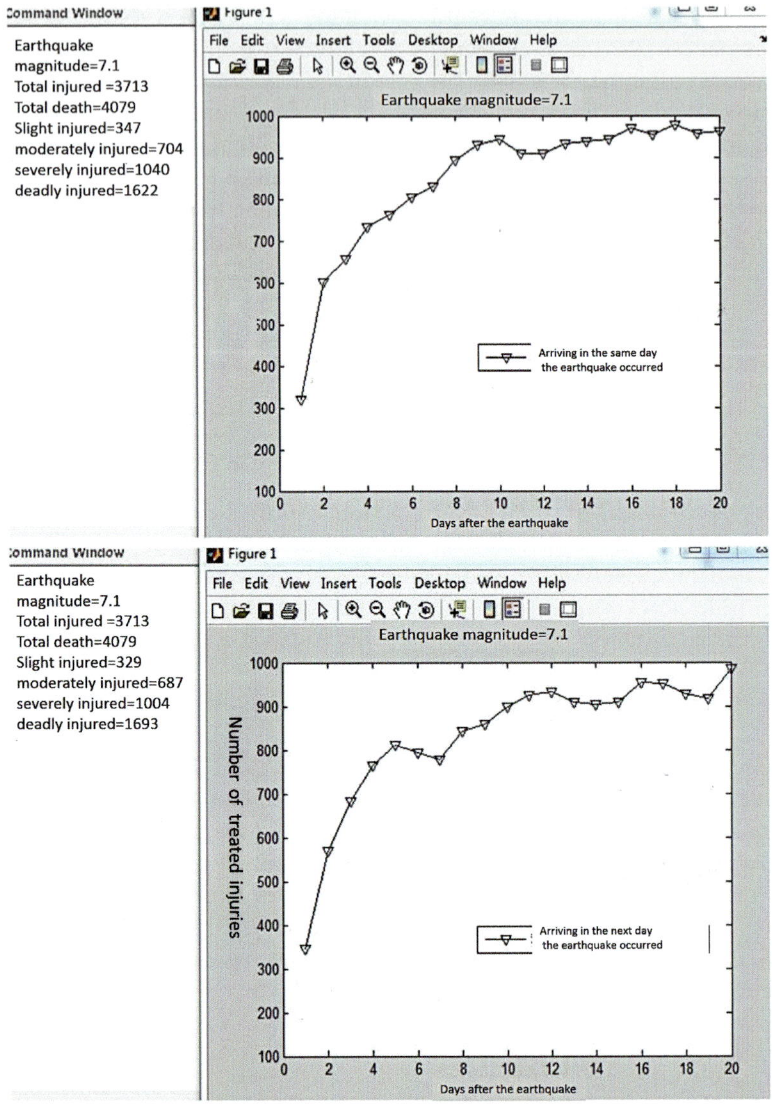

Fig. 2.6–2.8 Simulations of the model with different rescue speeds of outside support forces

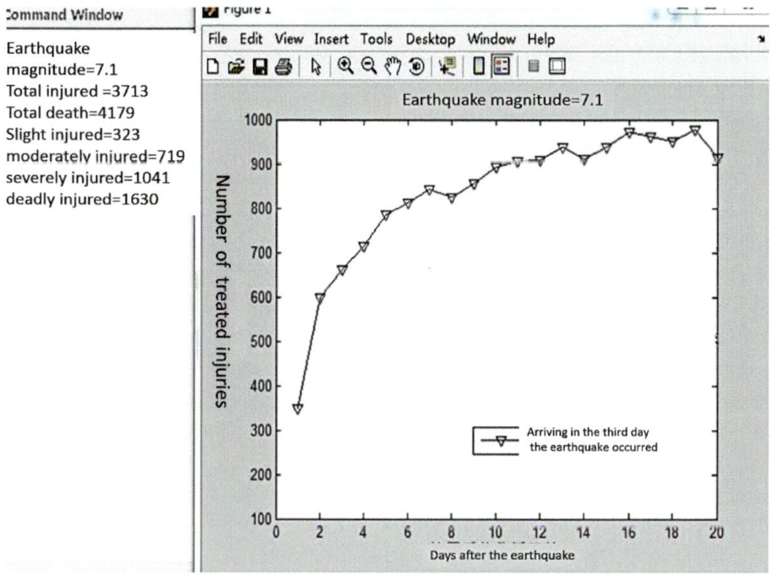

Fig. 2.6–2.8 (continued)

2.5 Summary

2.5.1 The Simulation of the Model Is Consistent with the Actual Occurrence of Casualties, Validating the "Two-Phase" Pattern

The model's simulations of the Yushu earthquake casualties were in line with the actual situation. In the simulation, the total number of injured was 17,295, the total number of deaths was 4186, the number of mildly injured persons was 7648, the number of moderately injured was 6741, the number of severely injured was 1802, and the number of deadly injured was 1104. The inflection point between the rapid growth period and the stable growth period was the sixth day after the Yushu earthquake. The actual number of injured was 12,135, the number of deaths was 2968, and the number of severely injured was 1434. The actual inflection point between the rapid growth period and the stable growth period was also the sixth day after the Yushu earthquake. Evidently, the model accurately simulated the casualty growth inflection point, and the orders of magnitude for the injured, dead, and severely injured were consistent between the simulation and the actual values. The deviation was 42.52 % for the injured, 41.04 % for the dead, and 23.01 % for the severely injured. The reasons for this discrepancy might be as follows: First, the model itself needs further adjustment; second, after the earthquake, the stricken area was in chaos and data collection did not accord with the actual situation—the deviation may have occurred when constructing the model with inaccurate data; and third, the impact of the medical relief staff in the modeling might have been derived from the delay caused by casualty evacuation. Thus, the model requires additional attention in future research.

The prediction trends of the injured being saved each day in the model were in line with the "two-phase" dynamic pattern. The inflection point emerged after the rapid growth period on the sixth day, after which the curve entered the stable growth period. After changing the earthquakes' magnitudes, the model's predictions found the following: When the earthquake magnitude was 5, the inflection point was the fourth day after the earthquake, and the first 4 day constituted the rapid growth period for casualties, after which the stable growth period emerged. When the magnitude was 6, the inflection point was the seventh day after the earthquake. For large-scale earthquakes (magnitude 8 or 9), the inflection point appeared later (both appearing on the eighth day in the prediction), and the curve is relatively smooth, with a long period of rapid growth and a less-obvious inflection point between the rapid and stable growth periods. These findings are in line with the influence of magnitude on the inflection point postulated by the "two-phase" dynamic pattern.

2.5.2 *The Model Predicts that Rescue Relief Arriving in the First Three Days is Crucial for Reducing Casualties*

Through analyzing the model simulations, it was found that whether all outside support forces arrived in the first 3 days after the earthquake had a significant impact on the medical treatment of the injured. Specifically, if the outside support medical forces arrived within the first 3 days, the total number of injured was only just over 3700, and the death toll was more than 4000, only 52 % of the actual casualties. This was much better than the actual situation. Within the first 3 days of the medical relief, the outside medical personnel arrived later, and the injury situation would deteriorate more quickly, with an increasing number of people dying. After the fifth day following the earthquake, the arrival of outside medical personnel could not prevent the deterioration of injury and death.

Therefore, the construction of the local earthquake medical relief forces, as well as the outside medical aid forces arriving in stricken areas within 24 h after earthquakes, could effectively reduce earthquake casualties and the severity of injuries and improve the prognosis for the injured.

References

Alexander D. On the spatial pattern of casualties in earthquakes. Ann Epidemiol. 2000;10(1):5–13.

Baitao S, Guixin Z. The Wenchuan earthquake creation of a rich database of building performance [J]. Sci China Technol Sci. 2010;53(10):2668–80.

China Earthquake Networks Center. http://www.csndmc.ac.cn/newweb/index.jsp.

Coburn AW. A Pomonis and S Sakai, assessing strategies to reduce fatalities in earthquakes, Proceedings of international workshop on earthquake injury Epidemiology for mitigation and response, July 10–12, 1989, Baltimore; 1989. p. 107–32.

Dezhi Y. Dictionary of earthquake,[M] Beijing, Seismological Press, 1990:250–74.

EM-DAT. Disaster List. 2000–10; Available from: http://www.emdat.be/search-details-disaster-list.

Garner A, Lee A, Harrison K, et al. Comparative analysis of multiple-casualty incident triage algorithms. Ann Emerg Med. 2001;38(5):541–8.

Gongxu G. China earthquake catalog (BC1831-AD1969). Beijing: Science Press; 1983.

Hamilton DR, Gavagan TF, Smart KT, et al. Houston's medical disaster response to Hurricane Katrina: part 1: the initial medical response from Trauma Service Area Q. Ann Emerg Med. 2009;53:505–14.

He Z, Guang F, Zhixiong T. Sichuan earthquake field hospital outpatient wounded disease spectrum analysis. Chinese Crit Care Med. 2008;28(9):796–9.

Hodgetts TJ, Mackway-Jones K. Major incident medical management and support. The practical approach. London: BMJ Publishing Group; 1995.

Hongfu C, Junwu D, Yanru W. Investigation report on influence factors of casualties in April14, 2010 Yushu earthquake. [J] Earthquake Engineering and Engineering Vibration. 2011;31(4): 18–25.

Jenkins JL, McCarthy ML, Sauer LM. Mass-casualty triage: time for an evidence-based approach. Prehospital Disaster Med. 2008;23(1):3–8.

Klain M, Semenov VN, Teriaev VG, et al. The results of resuscitation care in the earthquake in Armenia in 1988 [J]. Voen Med Zh. 1990;8:64–5.

Mulvey JM, Awan SU, Qadri AA. Profile of injuries arising from the 2005 Kashmir Earthquake: the first 72 h [J]. Injury Int J Care Injur. 2008;39:554–60.

Oike K. A discussion on the relation between magnitude and the number of the dead by earthquakes International seminar on earthquake prediction and hazard mitigation, technology, Japan, Science and Technology Agency. 1991.

Okada S. Indoor—zoning map on dwelling space safety during an earthquake. [A]. The Tenth World Conference on Earthquake Engineering[C]. Rotterdam: A. A Balkema; 1992. p. 6037–42.

On-Line CEU. Simple Triage and Rapid Transport (START) On-Line CEU for the Peoria Area EMS System and OSF Saint Francis Medical Center's ED Staff.

Pretto EA, Angus DC, Abrams JI, et al. Analysis of prehospital mortality in an earthquake. Disaster Reanimatology Study Group. PreHospital Disaster Med. 1994;9(2):107–17.

Qijia Z. The research of the loss of Chinese earthquake. In: Defense Secretary State Seismological Bureau damage future earthquake damage Research Group, Beijing: Earthquake Press; 1990.

Romig LE. Pediatric triage. A system to JumpSTART your triage of young patients at MCIs. [J] Jems J Emerg Med Serv. 2002;27(7):52–8, 60–3.

Schultz CH, Koenig KL. A medical disaster response to reduce immediate mortality after an earthquake. N Engl J Med. 1996;334(7):438–44.

Shiono K, Krimgold F, Ohta Y. Post-event rapid estimation of earthquake fatalities for the management of rescue activity. Comprehens Urban Stud. 1991;44:61–106.

Wang Y, Wang B, Junwu D. "5.12" Wenchuan earthquake spatial and temporal distribution of casualties [J]. J Nat Disasters. 2009;18(6):52–6.

Yanling Z. Non-war military operations duty health science. Beijing: People's Medical Publishing House; 2010.

Yehezkel W, Lisa A, Meirav M, et al. Prehospital response and field triage in pediatric mass casualty incidents: the Israeli experience. Clin Pediatr Emerg Med. 2006;7:52–8.

Yi Y. Natural disaster assessment study and practice progress [J]. Adv Earth Sci. 2010;25(1): 22–32.

Yokoyama H, Nagata S. A maze experiment of human behavior during evacuation [A] The Tenth World Conference on Earthquake Engineering [C]. Rotterdam: A. A. Balkema; 1992. p. 6061–9.

Zhang L, Liu X, Li Y, et al. Emergency medical rescue efforts after a major earthquake: lessons from the 2008 Wenchuan earthquake. Lancet. 2012;379(9818):853–61.

Zhao Z, Lin J, Zhong J. Earthquake casualties index and casualties state function [J]. J Nat Disasters. 1998;7(3):90–6.

Zhi B. The estimation of the spatial distribution of death caused by an earthquake [D]. Taiwan: National Central University; 2006.

Chapter 3
Logistic Regression Modeling for the Length of Stay Among the Hospitalized Patients After the 2010 Yushu Earthquake

Peng Kang and Lulu Zhang

Abstract *Objectives*: The aim was to identify factors that influence length of stay (LOS) among patients with earthquake-related injury and then to offer insights with respect to future directions for effective health policies and measures to reduce LOS.

Methods: This was a retrospective cohort study. Forty-nine rear hospitals spanning five provinces in China were included in the present study. Medical records of 2086 adult patients who were transported from the 2010 Yushu earthquake area and admitted for earthquake-related injury from April 14 to May 15, 2010, were collected.

Results: A total of 2086 patients with earthquake-related injury were included in this study, with a mean (SD) age of 40.0 (14.6) years. For comparative purposes, a longer LOS was defined as a hospital stay of over 25 days ($n=775$; 37.2 %), which represents the mean LOS value for all patients. Multivariate regression models show that being elderly (odds ratio [OR], 1.43; 95 % confidence interval [CI], 1.01–2.02), female (OR, 1.24; 95 % CI, 1.02–1.52), arriving earlier at the hospital (OR, 0.67; 95 % CI, 0.59–0.76), bone fracture (OR, 1.82; 95 % CI, 1.43–2.32), abdominal injury (OR, 1.62; 95 % CI, 1.20–2.17), injury to the extremities/pelvis injury (OR, 1.80; 95 % CI, 1.41–2.28), higher injury severity score (OR, 2.30; 95 % CI, 1.64–3.23), having undergone surgery (OR, 2.50; 95 % CI, 2.02–3.09), and having developed complications (OR, 1.74; 95 % CI, 1.20–2.54) were significantly and independently associated with longer LOS.

Conclusions: Strong preventive and therapeutic initiatives should be designed for elderly and female patients injured in earthquakes, especially within the initial days. Surgery was the greatest risk for a longer LOS. More attention should be paid to patients with fracture, trauma to the abdomen or extremities/pelvis, complications,

P. Kang, PhD
Faculty of Health Service, Institute of Military Health Management,
Second Military Medical University of the Chinese People's Liberation Army,
800 Xiangyin Road, Shanghai, People's Republic of China

L. Zhang, PhD (✉)
Department of Military Health Service, College of Military Health Service,
Second Military Medical University, Shanghai, China
e-mail: zllrmit@aliyun.com

© Springer Science+Business Media Dordrecht 2016

L. Zhang (ed.), *Modeling the Injury Flow and Treatment after Major Earthquakes*, DOI 10.1007/978-94-017-7527-4_3

or higher injury severity score. The factors identified in this study offer insights into directions for effective health policy to reduce LOS after a devastating earthquake.

3.1 Introduction

3.1.1 Background

3.1.1.1 Earthquake Disasters Are Serious in China, but Research on Injuries After Earthquakes Require Systematic Research

The ten most deadly earthquakes during the last century have killed more than 1.4 million people. Four of those earthquakes occurred in China and one each in Indonesia, Japan, the Soviet Union, Italy, Pakistan, and Haiti. Earthquakes affect human health directly by causing traumatic injuries and indirectly by disrupting healthcare systems. The dominant medical problem in the early phase after earthquakes is injuries. The early phase after earthquakes is characterized by chaos, and data collection is not a top priority. Thus, research on injuries due to earthquakes is lacking, and anecdotal reports from individual healthcare providers rather than systematic research dominate the literature.

3.1.1.2 The Yushu Earthquake Was Another Catastrophic Disaster Since the 2008 Wenchuan Earthquake that Involved a Substantial Number of Casualties

At 7:49 a.m. local time on April 14, 2010, a 7.1 magnitude earthquake struck Yushu prefecture in the Qinghai Province of China, which is located in a remote, high-altitude, mountainous region of the northeastern Tibetan Plateau (average elevation >4000 m). According to official records, the disaster killed 2698 and injured 12,135 people within an area of more than 20,000 km^2. Because the local medical care facilities were heavily damaged, transporting injured victims to rear hospitals in the early phase was common to decrease mortality and morbidity (Mulvey et al. 2008; Zhang et al. 2009). After the Yushu earthquake, a substantial number of victims with wounds and diseases were transported to peripheral hospitals spanning five provinces of China. This is known as the largest-scale evacuation of natural disaster victims from a high-altitude region in the history of our country.

3.1.1.3 Length of Hospital Stay Could Be an Important Factor in the Allocation of Medical Resources After Catastrophic Earthquakes

The ability to identify earthquake patients at risk for longer length of stay (LOS) may be valued by patients and policy makers. Risk stratification for LOS may help manage expectations regarding patient care and help to provide a means for identifying patients who will require additional attention and who may have more time for certain care strategies, including surgery and initiation of therapies. With the increased focus by Medicare and other organizations regarding readmissions, earthquake patients with expected shorter stays could potentially be triaged to short-stay observation units.

3.1.2 Current Situation and Literature Review

The current study was undertaken to identify predictors of hospital LOS for patients hospitalized with earthquake-related injury using clinical variables available at the time of admission and hospital characteristics. The hypothesis for this study was that certain patient characteristics would identify patients with shorter, intermediate, and longer LOS. In addition, the study tested whether there was incremental value in adding laboratory biomarker testing at the time of admission to predict LOS. LOS fulfills these criteria and has been validated as a precise proxy indicator for injury severity in non-disaster and high-income settings. However, there is less information regarding the factors influencing LOS among patients with earthquake-related injury, probably due to difficulties that hospitals might have with keeping complete and detailed medical records under chaotic conditions after a violent earthquake.

As a result, rear hospitals would receive a large number of injured patients in the initial days, and their treatment is often complex and costly, which undoubtedly make a considerable contribution to burden on hospitals (Fakhry et al. 2010). Effective healthcare resource management is especially indispensable for facilitating optimal use of scarce and critical healthcare resources (Finelli et al. 1989; Formiga et al. 2008). Hospital LOS, as an important outcome of inpatients, has received considerable attention. An increasing number of studies on the factors that determine LOS, or the capacity to predict an individual patient's LOS, have been performed in various specialty areas, ranging across various populations, such as the elderly (Formiga et al. 2008), adolescents (Sclar et al. 2008), and pregnant women (Moroy et al. 2007) to individuals with specific diseases/injuries, including heart failure (Formiga et al. 2008), malnutrition (Isabel et al. 2003), psychiatric issues (Wancata et al. 2001), burns (Yang et al. 2010), and fractures (Wilson and Stott 2007; Broadbent et al. 2010). A recent study focused on the predictors of hospital LOS in heart failure, finding that based on admission vital signs and BNP levels, patients with longer LOS have more comorbidities and higher disease severity. The ability to stratify risk for LOS based on patient admission and hospital characteristics is limited at present. Based on an empirical evaluation of 1080 burn cases collected in Taiwan, it was found that the accuracy of LOS predictions at the acute stage does not improve compared with those during the admission stage, but LOS predictions at the posttreatment stage are significantly more accurate. Moreover, artificial intelligence-based prediction techniques, especially support vector machine regression, appear more effective than the regression technique for LOS predictions for burn patients across stages. The target population included 322,894 discharges with a primary procedure code for primary total knee arthroplasty and 193,553 discharges for total hip arthroplasty. The variables associated with the greatest increases in length of stay were a higher comorbidity level among patient level attributes (+17.4 %) and low surgeon volume among provider-level characteristics (+18.8 %). Provider-level characteristics, particularly provider volume, had a greater impact on LOS. The presence of associated injuries was a key factor in initial LOS. However, the need for further operative interventions in the first hospital stay also increased LOS in some patients. Overall, the operative management of femoral fractures is resource intensive with a significant need for further minor operative intervention, regardless of the type of initial management. For 11 leading causes of acute hospital admissions in people aged >65 years, the National Health Service has generally lower hospital admission rates and longer hospital stays compared with Medicare recipients in the United States and California and Kaiser Permanente in California. More physician years in practice have been associated with less frequent guideline adherence, but it is unknown whether years in practice are associated with patient outcomes. Inpatient care by physicians with more years in practice is associated with higher risk of mortality. Quality-of-care interventions should be developed to maintain inpatient skills for physicians.

However, there is less information regarding the factors influencing LOS among patients with earthquake-related injury, likely due to the difficulties for hospitals in keeping complete and detailed medical records under chaotic conditions after a violent earthquake (Bulut et al. 2005).

3.1.3 Objective and Significance

3.1.3.1 Objective

The present study focused on patients hospitalized as a result of the 2010 Yushu earthquake and conducted comprehensive analyses on medical treatment received by the earthquake-related patients. Based on this situation, we also analyzed the LOS of patients and established the model of LOS.

3.1.3.2 Significance

The aim of this paper was to identify crucial factors influencing LOS among patients with earthquake-related injury based on the model established and then to offer insights into directions for effective health policies and clinical pathways formulated to reduce LOS.

3.2 Data Resource Used in the Model

3.2.1 Study Design

This study was approved and supported by the Chinese National Ministry of Health and the Health Department of Qinghai Province. We performed an external evaluation of the 2010 Yushu earthquake medical relief at the national level in December 2010. As part of the evaluation, we retrospectively analyzed inpatients with earthquake-related injury. Previous studies indicated the death in hospitals as a key variable for detecting factors related to death, and death has been demonstrated to be significantly associated with trauma, injury severity, various injuries, body region of injury, and complications. However, in the present study, among the 2086 earthquake-related patients of the Yushu earthquake, only four died due to extremely serious injuries after the earthquake, and all deaths occurred in the first 48 h after the earthquake. The mortality of hospitalized patients was only 0.1 %. Though the hospitalized death was a key variable in investigating patients hospitalized due to the earthquake, it could not account for the outcome of all hospitalized patients. Thus, hospital deaths were excluded from our study, and these cases were not identified in the research sample in the present study.

3.2.2 *Sampling and Data Collection*

A retrospective analysis of 2086 injured victims who were transported from the earthquake area and then admitted to 49 peripheral hospitals (including eight military hospitals) from April 14 to May 15, 2010, was included in the present study. Inclusion criteria included the following: adult patients (15 years or older), hospital admission within the first month following the earthquake, and earthquake-related injury as the cause of admission. Patient demographic data, complaints, diagnoses, injury types, disposition (including admission, discharge, and transfer), and means of transportation were individually reviewed according to the medical record database of each surveyed hospital. Patients who died during hospitalization or patients with incomplete medical data were excluded from the study. Double registrations were found for 213 patients who had been transferred to other hospitals for further treatment. To avoid repetition, duplicate records were combined into one record according to the patient's demographic data (Zhang et al. 2012).

3.2.3 *Definition of Variables*

Bivariate analyses were performed in order to identify the variables associated with longer LOS. The demographic and hospital admission variables included patient age, gender, means of transportation, and admission date. The importance of age as a predictor of patient outcomes was determined (Zhang et al. 2012; Perdue et al. 1998), and patients were divided into two groups: elderly (65 years or older) and younger patients (15–64 years old). Medical evacuation was defined as the transportation of the injured from the disaster area and into a higher-level treatment agency, not including transit within the disaster area or within hospitals. Means of evacuation were also classified into two categories: air transportation and land transportation.

We also included variables related to earthquake-related injury, preexisting diseases, surgery, and the development of complications. Injury types were determined based on final hospital diagnoses for injured patients as recorded by the attending physician. The injury sites were categorized based on the body region affected (head/neck, face, chest, abdomen/internal organs, extremities/pelvis, and body surface), and injury severity was identified by calculating an Injury Severity Score (ISS) based on the 2005 version of the Abbreviated Injury Scale (AIS-2005) (Osler et al. 1997; Foreman et al. 2007; Palmer et al. 2010).

3.2.4 Statistical Analysis

Descriptive statistics are reported as mean (± standard deviation, SD) for normally distributed continuous variables and as proportions for categorical variables. Student's *t*-test was used to evaluate differences in continuous variables, and the chi-squared test was used to assess associations between categorical variables. If continuous variables were not normally distributed, the Mann–Whitney *U*-test was applied. Bivariate and stepwise multivariate logistic regressions were used to identify the risk factors for longer LOS. All variables with $P<0.05$ in the bivariate analysis were entered into the multivariate models. The entry and removal criteria for the variables in the multivariate analysis were 0.05 and 0.10, respectively. $P<0.05$ was considered to be statistically significant. All statistical tests were two-tailed. Standard statistical software (SAS version 8.2) was used to perform all calculations.

3.3 Impact Factors of the Length of Stay Among Earthquake Patients

3.3.1 Descriptive Analysis

A total of 2086 adult patients were included in the study: 1080 males (51.8 %) and 1006 females. Their mean (range, SD) age was 40.0 (15–89, 14.6) years. The air evacuation system played an important role in the process of transferring injured victims to peripheral hospitals after the Yushu earthquake, with 87.8 % of injured patients being transported by air and 74.7 % being admitted within the initial 3 days following the earthquake. The most frequently occurring injuries were bone fractures, which were diagnosed in 1181 (56.6 %) patients. The lower extremities and pelvis (fractures, open wounds, and soft-tissue injuries) were the most frequently injured anatomical sites (36.0 %). Wound infection was the most common medical complication, followed by pneumonia and pulmonary edema. Consequently, 159 (7.6 %) hospitalized patients developed complications (Table 3.1).

Table 3.1 Description and bivariate analysis of demographic variables in both groups, according to the length of stay (LOS)

	Total	LOS ≤ 25 days	LOS > 25 days	
Variable	*n* (%)	(*n* = 1311)	(*n* = 775)	*p*-value
Age group				
Elderly	180 (8.6)	98 (7.5)	82 (10.6)	0.015
Younger adults	1906 (91.4)	1213 (92.5)	693 (89.4)	
Gender				
Male	1080 (51.8)	706 (53.9)	374 (48.3)	0.014
Female	1006 (48.2)	605 (46.1)	401 (51.7)	
Means of evacuation				
By air	1832 (87.8)	1154 (88.0)	678 (87.5)	0.715
By ground	254 (12.2)	157 (12.0)	97 (12.5)	
Days between injury and admission				
≤1 day	474 (22.7)	245 (18.7)	229 (29.6)	0.03
2–3 days	1085 (52.0)	653 (49.8)	432 (55.7)	
4–7 days	364 (17.5)	279 (21.3)	85 (11.0)	
>7 days	163 (7.8)	134 (10.2)	29 (3.7)	

3.3.2 *Bivariate Analysis*

3.3.2.1 Overall Analysis of Length of Stay

A mean (range, SD) LOS of 24.7 (1–203, 18.2) days for the entire patient population indicated substantial resource consumption. Overall, 775 patients (37.2 %) experienced an LOS longer than 25 days, and 1131 patients experienced a shorter stay (≤25 days). Further, 23 patients (1.1 %) experienced an LOS longer than 3 months.

3.3.2.2 Bivariate Analysis

Bivariate analysis was used to explore the effect of selected variables on longer LOS. Table 3.1 shows that a significant increase in LOS was found among adults who were elderly ($p = 0.015$) and female ($p = 0.014$). Unexpectedly, a negative association was observed for admission date, which indicates that those who were admitted to hospitals earlier were more likely to experience a longer LOS. As seen in Table 3.2, a longer LOS was also associated with several injury-specific characteristics as follows: suffering from bone fractures, abdominal injuries, extremity/pelvis injuries, higher ISS, a maximal AIS, several body regions injured, preexisting diseases, the development of complications, and having undergone surgery.

Table 3.2 Description and bivariate analysis of earthquake-related injury variables in both groups according to length of stay (LOS)

Variable	Total	LOS $\leq$ 25 days (n = 1311)	LOS > 25 days (n = 775)	p-value
Injury type				
Fracture	1181 (56.6)	597 (45.5)	585 (75.5)	<0.001
Multiple soft-tissue contusion	534 (25.6)	405 (30.9)	129 (16.7)	<0.001
Open or closed wound	668 (32.0)	468 (35.7)	200 (25.8)	<0.001
Crush injuries	72 (3.5)	48 (3.7)	24 (3.1)	0.495
Burn and scald	206 (9.9)	127 (9.7)	79 (10.2)	0.708
Other injuries	63 (3.0)	42 (3.2)	21 (2.7)	0.524
Injured body site				
Head/neck	206 (9.9)	153 (11.7)	5.3 (6.8)	<0.001
Face	120 (5.8)	84 (6.4)	36 (4.7)	0.095
Thorax	385 (18.5)	223 (17.0)	162 (20.9)	0.027
Abdomen/internal organs	324 (15.5)	163 (12.4)	161 (20.8)	<0.001
Extremities and pelvis	969 (46.5)	475 (36.2)	494 (63.7)	<0.001
External	754 (36.1)	540 (41.2)	214 (27.6)	<0.001
Injury severity score	5.4 ± 5.1	4.3 ± 3.9	7.3 ± 6.3	<0.001
Maximal abbreviated injury score	2.0 ± 0.8	1.8 ± 0.7	2.3 ± 0.9	<0.001
Number of body regions injured	1.3 ± 0.6	1.2 ± 0.5	1.4 ± 0.7	<0.001
Preexisting diseases	123 (5.9)	64 (4.9)	59 (7.6)	0.011
Having developed complications	159 (7.6)	72 (5.5)	87 (11.2)	<0.001
Having been performed surgery	732 (35.1)	301 (23.0)	431 (55.6)	<0.001

Values are expressed as the number (percentage) or mean ± standard derivation

Table 3.3 Risk factors for a longer length of stay in the patient population

Variable	Odds ratio	95 % CI	p-value
Being elderly (≥65 years old)	1.43	1.01–2.02	0.044
Days between injury and admission[a]	0.67	0.59–0.76	<0.001
Gender (female)	1.24	1.02–1.52	0.036
Having developed complications	1.74	1.20–2.54	0.004
Bone fracture	1.82	1.43–2.32	<0.001
Abdomen/pelvis contents injury	1.62	1.20–2.17	0.001
Extremities and pelvis injury	1.8	1.41–2.28	<0.001
Having been performed surgery	2.5	2.02–3.09	<0.002
Injury severity score	2.3	1.64–3.23	<0.003

[a]≤1 day = 1, 2–3 days = 2, 4–7 days = 3, >7 days = 4. *CI* confidence interval

3.4 Modeling and Analysis of Length of Stay Among Hospitalized Patients

3.4.1 Constructing the Model of Length of Stay Among Hospitalized Patients

In the present study, hospital LOS was considered as the dependent variable, and associations between longer LOS and values of explanatory variables were explored in earthquake-injury patients. LOS was defined as the total number of days spent in the hospital. For comparative purposes, a longer LOS was defined as a hospital stay of over 25 days ($n=775$; 37.2 %), which represents the mean LOS value for all patients. We also included variables related to demographics, admission information, earthquake-related injury, preexisting diseases, surgery, and the development of complications. The injury sites were categorized based on the body region affected (head/neck, face, chest, abdomen/internal organs, extremities/pelvis, and body surface), and the severity of injury was identified by calculating an ISS based on the AIS-2005. All variables with $P<0.05$ in the bivariate analysis were entered into the multivariate models. Standard statistical software (SAS version 8.2) was used to perform all calculations. The logistic model was established as follows:

$$Logit(P) = y = 62.2973 - 2.3133X_1 - 2.2447X_2 + 1.4493X_3 + 2.0676X_4 - \\ 4.7238X_5 - 3.5160X_6 - 5.4045X_7 + 1.4493X_8 + 2.0676X_9 - 4.7238X_{10}, \\ \left(F = 38.64, p < 0.0001, R^2 = 0.5529\right)$$

Table 3.3 shows the results of the multivariable logistic regression analysis. Being elderly (odds ratio (OR)=1.43, 95 % confidence interval (CI): 1.01–2.02), female (OR=1.24, 95 % CI: 1.02–1.52), arriving earlier at the hospital (OR=0.67, 95 % CI: 0.59–0.76), bone fractures (OR=1.82, 95 % CI: 1.43–2.32), injury to the abdomen (OR=1.62, 95 % CI: 1.20–2.17), injury to the extremities/pelvis (OR=1.80, 95 % CI: 1.41–2.28), higher ISS (OR=2.30, 95 % CI: 1.64–3.23), having undergone surgery (OR=2.50, 95 % CI: 2.02–3.09), and having developed complications (OR=1.74, 95 % CI: 1.20–2.54) were significantly and independently associated with LOS longer than 25 days.

3.4.2 Analysis of Impact Factors of Length of Stay Among Hospitalized Patients

3.4.2.1 The Key Reasons for Low Mortality

In the present study, hospital LOS was considered as the dependent variable, and associations between longer LOS and values of explanatory variables were explored among earthquake-injury patients. As seen in other studies, however, mortality was also chosen as a major outcome (Peek-Asa et al. 1998; Perdue et al. 1998), and survival after trauma was demonstrated to be related to injury severity, type of trauma, and complications that developed (Horst et al. 1986). In our study, the hospital mortality rate was extremely low (0.1 %), with only three patients dying while in the hospital. Deaths were excluded from our study because all of them occurred within 48 h after admission. This low mortality rate may reflect the effective relief work organized by the Chinese government. In addition, the intensity of the earthquake and the local demographics were important factors. The Yushu earthquake was relatively low in magnitude and intensity compared to the 1976 Tangshan earthquake (7.8 on the Richter scale) and the 2008 Wenchuan earthquake (8.0 on the Richter scale). In addition, the disaster occurred in a sparsely populated area on the plateau. Although survival is a clear-cut, easily measurable outcome, it is not an applicable outcome to accurately capture the consequences of injury in our study. Thus, we chose the mean LOS of our cohort as the cut-off point for differentiating a longer LOS, which has been frequently used in previous studies (Wright et al. 2003; Formiga et al. 2008; Tamim et al. 2008). However, our patients' mean LOS was considerably longer than that reported in previous studies on patients with specific diseases (Richmond et al. 2002; Formiga et al. 2008), likely because of the fact that earthquake-related injuries can be much more severe and may require more specific care.

3.4.2.2 Demographic Contributors to Length of Stay

Previous studies have discussed the effects of serious injury among elderly patients (65 years or older) (Horst et al. 1986; Finelli et al. 1989; Richmond et al. 2002). Due to physiologic changes including decreased bone mass, diminished fat stores, loss of subcutaneous tissue, and muscle atrophy, elderly individuals tolerate earthquake-related injury less effectively than younger patients do (Knudson et al. 1994; Erek et al. 2001). Traumatic injury in elderly adults is more complex and severe, and considerable healthcare resources are required to manage seriously injured older adults (Richmond et al. 2002). In the present study, elderly patients experienced a longer LOS in comparison to younger ones (45.6 % vs. 36.4 %), and being elderly was also implicated as a cause of mortality among trauma patients in other studies (Horst et al. 1986). Gender represents another important factor. Our finding of an association between being female and longer LOS supports previous studies (Babiker 1980; Kastrup 1987; Jakubas chk et al. 1993). Formiga et al. (2008) found that female gender was one of only two significant factors independently associated with longer LOS (Formiga et al. 2008). One hypothesis to explain this association might be that women moved slower than men did to avoid falling objects during the earthquake, as well as lower tolerance to earthquake-related injuries. Taken together, an examination of the injuries in elderly and female patients following a devastating earthquake is worthy of more attention. Developing interventions targeted toward elderly and female patients may also help to decrease LOS.

3.4.2.3 Medical Evacuation Contributes to Length of Stay

Air evacuation has been widely used in earthquake relief works worldwide (Tanaka et al. 1998). Previous studies have demonstrated the merits of medical airlifts for injuries, as this could lead to a 21–52 % decrease in mortality, especially for traumatized patients (Baxt and Moody 1983; Baxt et al. 1985). Air evacuation played an important role in the transfer of injured victims after the Yushu earthquake for several reasons. First, Yushu prefecture is located in a remote, high-altitude region, and roads to the epicentral area were seriously damaged (Tie-Min 2010). Second, the nearest city (Chengdu) is almost 490 km from the Yushu prefecture. Third, the Batang airport, which is only 18 km away, was first put into use in August 2009 and facilitated timely air transportation. Although air evacuation was used to transport approximately 70 % of the patients admitted within the initial 3 days after the earthquake from the plateau, the present study did not find an association between the means of evacuation and LOS. The first 72 h after an earthquake is considered to be the "golden relief time" for rescue because the chances of survival improve with reduced times to evacuation. Our findings showed that patients who arrived at the hospital earlier tended to experience a longer LOS. One possible reason is that the triage work was performed effectively in the earthquake area and that victims with severe injuries had to be transported to peripheral hospitals for further treatment. This finding suggests that greater attention and more specific treatment are required in treating injured victims hospitalized during the initial days following an earthquake.

3.4.2.4 Earthquake-Related Injury Contributes to Length of Stay

Earthquakes, which cause a significant loss of life and a dramatic increase in the incidence of complex injuries in victims, are known as the most unpredictable and hazardous type of disaster (Reitherman 1986; Binder and Sanderson 1987; Mahoney and Reutershan 1987; Mulvey et al. 2008). Tanaka et al. (1999) found that fractures constituted 54.8 % of all the injuries following the 1995 Hanshin-Awaji earthquake, with extremity fractures being the most common (37.2 %). Similar injury patterns were also found after the 1994 Northridge earthquake (Peek-Asa et al. 1998). Our results are consistent with these findings. Tanaka et al. (1999) also reported that cranial, thoracic, and abdominal injuries were associated with mortality among these cases. Among the injury-specific variables in the present study, bone fracture (OR = 1.82), injury to abdominal organs (OR = 1.62), and injury to the extremities or pelvis (OR = 1.80) increased the odds of a longer LOS. ISS has been widely used as an indicator of injury severity and a predictor of patient outcome, and Tamim et al. (2008) reported that the ISS is superior to other scoring systems in predicting LOS. However, other studies have reported that ISS is a poor predictor of outcomes in elderly adults (Horst et al. 1986; Pudelek 2002). The present study was performed among earthquake-related trauma patients and found that the ISS is a significant predictor of longer LOS.

3.4.2.5 Surgical Procedures and Complications Contribute to Length of Stay

Resource utilization after surgical procedures can escalate dramatically when complications arise, particularly in the subsequent postoperative intensive care unit recovery period (Rowan et al. 2007). The present study also indicated that surgery was the greatest risk for longer LOS (OR = 2.50) among all variables in the multivariate model. It is not surprising that trauma patients who have undergone surgery require more medical care and require a longer LOS. Kim (2011) also demonstrated that when brain-injured patients undergo surgery within 4 h of emergency department arrival, their LOS is significantly shorter. Therefore, early surgery and identification of patients at greater risk of developing postoperative complications could promote the development of efficient clinical pathways and optimization of healthcare resource management (Doering et al. 2001).

This study also demonstrated that the most common medical complication is wound infection among earthquake inpatients, followed by pneumonia, similar to findings after the 2008 Wenchuan earthquake (Zhang et al. 2012). Although a relatively small number of injured patients in our study experienced complications, the presence of any complication significantly increases the odds of experiencing a longer LOS. This result was consistent with the previous studies in unselected groups of patients (Iezzoni et al. 1994) and in those hospitalized for stroke rehabilitation (Brosseau et al. 1996). Richard et al. also reported that subsequent hospital complications, including pressure ulcers, infections, and other incident complications, were predictive of total cost and suggested that interventions established to prevent hospital complications merit evaluation as ways to decrease hospital LOS and costs (Allman et al. 1999). Previous studies also demonstrated that preexisting medical diseases were associated with death after trauma (Pickering et al. 1999; Tepas III et al. 2000). In the present study, preexisting diseases did not contribute to a longer LOS.

3.4.2.6 Study Limitations

To the best of our knowledge, the present study is the first to explore the factors that influence hospital LOS among a large number of injured patients after a devastating earthquake on the national level. However, there are also notable limitations to our study. First, the analysis did not assess the impact of physiological parameters on LOS. The detailed medical records of all hospitalized patients were often incomplete because of initial disorganization, especially during the first few hours after the earthquake (Bulut et al. 2005). Second, our study utilized a retrospective design. Although most epidemiological studies of earthquake patients rely on the medical records of surveyed hospitals (Peek-Asa et al. 1998; Bulut et al. 2005; Zhang et al. 2012), the variables used in formulating intervention strategies should be collected concurrently to ultimately improve outcomes (Richmond et al. 2002). Third, our study failed to consider the impact of medical treatment choices on LOS. Our study only examined the impact of surgery, as in-hospital management choices were complex and varied across hospitals.

3.5 Summary

The aim was to identify factors that influence LOS among patients with earthquake-related injury and then to offer insights with respect to future directions for effective health policies and measures to reduce LOS. Participants in the study were adult patients who were transported from the 2010 Yushu earthquake area and admitted for earthquake-related injury from April 14 to May 15, 2010. LOS was defined as the total number of days spent in the hospital. For comparative purposes, a longer LOS was defined as a hospital stay of over 25 days ($n = 775$; 37.2 %), which represents the mean LOS value for all patients. Descriptive statistics and bivariate and stepwise multivariate logistic regressions were used to identify risk factors for longer LOS.

3.5.1 The Proportion of Males Was Significantly Higher Than that of Females, and the Air Evacuation System Played An Important Role

A total of 2086 adult patients were included in the study. The air evacuation system played an important role in the process of transferring injured victims to peripheral hospitals, with 87.8 % of injured patients being transported by air and 74.7 % being admitted within the initial 3 days following the earthquake. The most frequently occurring injuries were bone fractures. The lower extremities and pelvis (fractures, open wounds, and soft-tissue injuries) were the most frequently injured anatomical sites (36.0 %). Wound infection was the most common medical complication.

3.5.2 The Mean (Range, SD) Length of Stay Was 24.7 (1–203, 18.2) Days, and 23 Patients (1.1 %) Experienced an LOS Longer Than 3 Months

A mean (range, SD) LOS of 24.7 (1–203, 18.2) days for the entire patient population indicated substantial resource consumption. Overall, 775 patients (37.2 %) experienced an LOS longer than 25 days, and 1131 patients experienced a shorter stay (≤25 days). Further, 23 patients (1.1 %) experienced an LOS longer than 3 months.

3.5.3 *Patients Who Were Elderly, Were Female, Had Bone Fractures, and Had Undergone Surgery Associated with Several Injury-Specific Characteristics*

Bivariate analysis showed a significant increase in LOS among adults who were elderly and female. Unexpectedly, a negative association was observed for admission date in the present study, indicating that those who were admitted to hospitals earlier were more likely to experience a longer LOS. A longer LOS was also associated with several injury-specific characteristics as follows: suffering from bone fractures, abdominal injuries, extremity/pelvis injuries, higher ISS, a maximal AIS, several body regions injured, preexisting diseases, the development of complications, and having undergone surgery.

3.5.4 *The Factors Identified in This Study Offer Insights Into Directions for Effective Health Policy to Reduce LOS After a Devastating Earthquake*

Being elderly, female, number of days between injury and admission, bone fractures, injury to the abdomen, injury to the extremities/pelvis, higher ISS, having undergone surgery, and having developed complications were significantly and independently associated with LOS longer than 25 days. Strong preventive and therapeutic initiatives should be designed for elderly and female patients injured in earthquakes, especially within the initial days. Surgery was the greatest risk for a longer LOS. More attention should be paid to the patients with fracture, trauma to the abdomen or trauma to the extremities/pelvis, complications, and higher ISS.

Therefore, strong preventive and therapeutic initiatives should be designed for high-risk patients injured in earthquakes, especially within the initial days. The factors identified in this study offer insights into directions for effective health policy to reduce LOS after a devastating earthquake.

References

Allman RM, et al. Pressure ulcers, hospital complications, and disease severity: impact on hospital costs and length of stay. Adv Wound Care: J Prevent Heal. 1999;12(1):22. ISSN 1076-2191.

Babiker IE. Social and clinical correlates of the 'new'long – stay. Acta Psychiatrica Scandinavica. 1980;61(4):365–75. ISSN 1600-0447.

Baxt WG, Moody P. The impact of a rotorcraft aeromedical emergency care service on trauma mortality. JAMA. 1983;249(22):3047. ISSN 0098-7484.

Baxt WG, et al. Hospital-based rotorcraft aeromedical emergency care services and trauma mortality: a multicenter study. Ann Emerg Med. 1985;14(9):859–64. ISSN 0196-0644.

Binder S, Sanderson LM. The role of the epidemiologist in natural disasters. Ann Emerg Med. 1987;16(9):1081–4. ISSN 0196-0644.

Broadbent MR, Will E, Mcqueen MM. Prediction of outcome after humeral diaphyseal fracture. Injury. 2010;41(6):572–7. ISSN 00201383.

Brosseau L, et al. Post-stroke inpatient rehabilitation. I. Predicting length of stay. Am J Phys Med Rehabil. 1996; 75(6):422–30. ISSN 0894-9115 (Print) 0894-9115 (Linking). Available at: http://www.ncbi.nlm.nih.gov/pubmed/8985105.

Bulut M, et al. Medical experience of a university hospital in Turkey after the 1999 Marmara earthquake. Emerg Med J. 2005;22(7):494. ISSN 1472-0213.

Doering LV, et al. Determinants of intensive care unit length of stay after coronary artery bypass graft surgery. Heart Lung. 2001;30(1):9–17. ISSN 0147-9563 (Print) 0147-9563 (Linking). Available at: http://www.ncbi.nlm.nih.gov/pubmed/11174363.

Erek E, et al. The Marmara earthquake: epidemiological analysis of the victims with nephrological problems. Kidney Int. 2001;60(3):1114–23. ISSN 0085-2538.

Fakhry SM, et al. Trauma center finances and length of stay: identifying a profitability inflection point. J Am Coll Surg. 2010;210(5):817–21. ISSN 10727515.

Finelli FC, et al. A case control study for major trauma in geriatric patients. J Trauma. 1989;29(5):541. ISSN 0022-5282.

Foreman BP, et al. Usefulness of the abbreviated injury score and the injury severity score in comparison to the Glasgow Coma Scale in predicting outcome after traumatic brain injury. J Trauma. 2007;62(4):946. ISSN 0022-5282.

Formiga F, Chivite D, Manito N, et al. Admission characteristics predicting longer length of stay among elderly patients hospitalized for decompensated heart failure [J]. Eur J Int Med. 2008;19(3):198–202. ISSN 0953-6205. Available at: http://www.sciencedirect.com/science/article/pii/S095362050700266X.

Horst HM, et al. Factors influencing survival of elderly trauma patients. Crit Care Med. 1986;14(8):681. ISSN 0090-3493.

Iezzoni LI, et al. Identifying complications of care using administrative data. Med Care 1994;32(7):700–151994. ISSN 0025-7079 (Print) 0025-7079 (Linking). Available at: http://www.ncbi.nlm.nih.gov/pubmed/8028405.

Isabel TD, Correia M. The impact of malnutrition on morbidity, mortality, length of hospital stay and costs evaluated through a multivariate model analysis. Clin Nutr. 2003;22(3):235–9. ISSN 02615614.

Jakubaschk J, Waldvogel D, Würmle O. Differences between long-stay and short-stay inpatients and estimation of length of stay. Soc Psychiatr Psychiatr Epidemiol. 1993;28(2):84–90. ISSN 0933-7954.

Kastrup M. Prediction and profile of the long – stay population. Acta Psychiatrica Scandinavica. 1987;76(1):71–9. ISSN 1600-0447.

Kim YJ. The impact of time from ED arrival to surgery on mortality and hospital length of stay in patients with traumatic brain injury. J Emer Nurs. 2011;37(4):328–33. ISSN 00991767.

Knudson MM, et al. Mortality factors in geriatric blunt trauma patients. Arch Surg. 1994;129(4):448.

Mahoney LE, Reutershan TP. Catastrophic disasters and the design of disaster medical care systems. Ann Emerg Med. 1987;16(9):1085–91. ISSN 0196-0644.

Moroy P, et al. Factors influencing the postpartum length of hospital stay in eclamptic women. Taiwanese J Obst Gynecol. 2007;46(4):410–3. ISSN 10284559.

Mulvey J, et al. Profile of injuries arising from the 2005 Kashmir earthquake: the first 72 h. Injury. 2008;39(5):554–60. ISSN 0020-1383.

Osler T, Baker SP, Long W. A modification of the injury severity score that both improves accuracy and simplifies scoring. J Trauma. 1997;43(6):922. ISSN 0022-5282.

Palmer CS, Niggemeyer LE, Charman D. Double coding and mapping using Abbreviated Injury Scale 1998 and 2005: Identifying issues for trauma data. Injury. 2010;41(9):948–54. ISSN 0020-1383.

Peek-Asa C, et al. Fatal and hospitalized injuries resulting from the 1994 Northridge earthquake. Int J Epidemiol. 1998;27(3):459. ISSN 0300-5771.

Perdue PW, et al. Differences in mortality between elderly and younger adult trauma patients: geriatric status increases risk of delayed death. J Trauma. 1998;45(4):805. ISSN 0022-5282.

Pickering S, Esberger D, Moran C. The outcome following major trauma in the elderly. Predictors of survival. Injury. 1999;30(10):703–6. ISSN 0020-1383.

Pudelek B. Geriatric trauma: special needs for a special population. AACN Adv Crit Care. 2002;13(1):61. ISSN 1559-7768.

Reitherman R. How to prepare a hospital for an earthquake. J Emerg Med. 1986;4(2):119–31. ISSN 0736-4679.

Richmond TS, et al. Characteristics and outcomes of serious traumatic injury in older adults. J Am Geriatr Soc. 2002;50(2):215–22. ISSN 1532-5415.

Rowan M, et al. The use of artificial neural networks to stratify the length of stay of cardiac patients based on preoperative and initial postoperative factors. Artif Intell Med. 2007;40(3):211–21. ISSN 09333657.

Sclar DA, et al. Hospital length of stay for children and adolescents diagnosed with depression: is primary payer an influencing factor? Gen Hosp Psychiatr. 2008;30(1):73–6. ISSN 01638343.

Tamim H, et al. The injury severity score or the new injury severity score for predicting mortality, intensive care unit admission and length of hospital stay: experience from a university hospital in a developing country. Injury. 2008;39(1):115–20. ISSN 00201383.

Tanaka H, et al. Overview of evacuation and transport of patients following the 1995 Hanshin-Awaji earthquake 1 2. J Emerg Med. 1998;16(3):439–44. ISSN 0736-4679.

Tanaka H, et al. Morbidity and mortality of hospitalized patients after the 1995 Hanshin-Awaji earthquake. Am J Emerg Med. 1999;17(2):186–91. ISSN 0735-6757.

Tepas III JJ, et al. Elderly injury: a profile of trauma experience in the Sunshine (Retirement) State. J Trauma. 2000;48(4):581. ISSN 0022-5282.

Tie-Min L. The significance of emergency preparedness highlighted by Yushu earthquake once again [J]. J Saf Sci Technol. 2010;2:003.

Wancata J, Benda N, Windhaber J, et al. Does psychiatric comorbidity increase the length of stay in general hospitals? [J]. Gen Hosp Psychiatr. 2001;23(1):8–14.

Wilson NC, Stott NS. Paediatric femoral fractures: Factors influencing length of stay and readmission rate. Injury. 2007;38(8):931–6. ISSN 0020-1383. Available at: http://www.sciencedirect.com/science/article/pii/S0020138307001246.

Wright S, et al. Factors influencing the length of hospital stay of patients with heart failure. Eur J Heart Fail. 2003;5(2):201–9. ISSN 1388-9842.

Yang C-S, et al. Predicting the length of hospital stay of burn patients: Comparisons of prediction accuracy among different clinical stages. Decision Suppt Syst. 2010;50(1):325–35. ISSN 0167-9236. Available at: http://www.sciencedirect.com/science/article/pii/S0167923610001703.

Zhang L, et al. The injury profile after the 2008 earthquakes in China. Injury. 2009;40(1):84–6. ISSN 0020-1383.

Zhang L, Fu P, Wang L, et al. The clinical features and outcome of crush patients with acute kidney injury after the Wenchuan earthquake: differences between elderly and younger adults [J]. Injury. 2012;43(9):1470–75. ISSN 0020-1383. Available at: http://www.sciencedirect.com/science/article/pii/S0020138310007734.

Chapter 4
Modeling Earthquake-Related Medical Evacuation

Xu Liu, Hongyang Yang, Haiping Chen, and Lulu Zhang

Abstract Our research group first discovered that emergency medical rescue could be divided into "two periods and three stages" during an empirical study of the Wenchuan earthquake emergency medical rescue. According to this framework of "two periods," the "increasing period" began directly after the earthquake and continued for 1–2 weeks. During it, the number of patients needing emergency medical attention increased. For the first 72 h after the earthquake, rescue work was in an "emergency stage." The medical service system in the disaster areas was paralyzed, and the majority of supporting medical rescue power did not arrive. Therefore, first-line treatment ability could not match the treatment needs of patients in the disaster areas, so patients' medical evacuation became a priority. In general, there are two main strategies used in emergency medical rescue after major earthquakes. One is the mobilization of a large number of elite medical resources such as field hospitals, forward surgical teams, and medical specialists who rush to the front line of the disaster areas. The other is the evacuation of patients from the disaster site after a simple triage to rear echelon hospitals in unaffected areas for definitive treatment. In this chapter, we show that medical evacuation research about earthquake patients mainly indicates that patients flow from the disaster areas to the rear hospitals for specialized treatment within the "increasing period," corresponding "emergency stage," and "effective stage".

X. Liu • H. Chen
Department of Military Health Service, College of Military Health Service, Second Military Medical University, Yangpu, Shanghai, China

H. Yang, PhD
The General Hospital of the PLA Rocket Force, Yangpu, Shanghai, China

L. Zhang, PhD (✉)
Department of Military Health Service, College of Military Health Service, Second Military Medical University, Shanghai, China
e-mail: zllrmit@aliyun.com

© Springer Science+Business Media Dordrecht 2016
L. Zhang (ed.), *Modeling the Injury Flow and Treatment after Major Earthquakes*, DOI 10.1007/978-94-017-7527-4_4

4.1 An Introduction to Earthquake Medical Evacuation

4.1.1 Background

4.1.1.1 A Patient Medical Evacuation System Is a Core Component of the "Two Periods and Three Stages" of Emergency Medical Rescue

Our research group first discovered that emergency medical rescue could be divided into "two periods and three stages" during an empirical study of the Wenchuan earthquake emergency medical rescue. According to this framework of "two periods," the "increasing period" began directly after the earthquake and continued for 1–2 weeks. During it, the number of patients needing emergency medical attention increased. For the first 72 h after the earthquake, rescue work was in an "emergency stage." The medical service system in the disaster areas was paralyzed, and the majority of supporting medical rescue power did not arrive. Therefore, first-line treatment ability could not match the treatment needs of patients in the disaster areas, so patients' medical evacuation became a priority. In general, there are two main strategies used in emergency medical rescue after major earthquakes. One is the mobilization of a large number of elite medical resources such as field hospitals, forward surgical teams, and medical specialists who rush to the front line of the disaster areas. The other is the evacuation of patients from the disaster site after a simple triage to rear echelon hospitals in unaffected areas for definitive treatment. In this chapter, we show that medical evacuation research about earthquake patients mainly indicates that patients flow from the disaster areas to the rear hospitals for specialized treatment within the "increasing period," corresponding "emergency stage," and "effective stage".

4.1.1.2 How the Efficiency of Evacuation Was Directly Influenced by the Structural Barriers of the Patients' Medical Evacuation System

The large scale of the Wenchuan and Yushu earthquakes, their sudden occurrence, the complex injuries sustained by people, and the damage wrought upon transportation, communication, and power systems raised major challenges for the evacuation of patients. The rescue work of Wenchuan earthquake and Yushu earthquake indicated that disorder and blind mind rescue not only waste resources but also put weight on difficulty of treatment. In the Wenchuan rescue, a number of specialized medical personnel gathered on the front line of the disaster areas. Due to the lack of power, equipment, and treatment conditions, they (particularly the neurosurgeons, urology surgeons, and thoracic surgeons) could not carry out specialized, on-site treatment. On the contrary, hospitals near the disaster area with a heavy treatment load needed a large number of high-quality medical rescue resources. Setting up an appropriate evacuation standard and deploying proper medical rescue resources according to echelon treatment turned into the key for improving the efficiency of medical evacuation.

4.1.1.3 An Earthquake Medical Evacuation System Is a Typically Complex Adaptive System

Uncertainty about an earthquake's arrival time, location, intensity, scale, and the damage it could cause to transportation, the environment, and communication provokes chaos within a region or even a country undergoing an "emergency stage." An earthquake medical evacuation system must take into account the disaster areas, each evacuation echelon, and rear hospitals, and it must address the needs of patients, medical personnel, and decision makers. Military, police, civilians, logistics, and transportation have to be coordinated. The environment is often complicated, too, by a lack of resources. All of these features suggest that an earthquake evacuation system is a typically complex adaptive system. Scientific discussion about evacuation is particularly important, and having a reasonable treatment echelon, appropriate rear hospitals, and evacuating vehicles is related to the effects of evacuation.

4.1.2 Current Situation and Literature Review

4.1.2.1 Review of the Medical Evacuation Process After the Wenchuan and Yushu Earthquakes

Evacuation System

The evacuation system put in place after the Wenchuan earthquake had the following characteristics: evacuation to nearby hospitals, bypassing the immediate evacuation echelon, combining military and civilian hospitals, and establishing trans-provincial evacuation. Overall, evacuations were carried out in three steps. The first step included transporting patients on the spot to nearby hospitals in the hardest-hit disaster area. The second step was triaging and shunting patients who were stranded at the medical station in the hardest-hit disaster areas and transporting those who needed further treatment to hospitals outside of the disaster areas. The third step was a process trans-provincial evacuation, which sent patients nationwide. Overall, 10,015 patients were transported to 375 hospitals in 58 cities and 20 provinces (Chen et al. 2009; Xu et al. 2009; Zhang et al. 2012).

The evacuation system that was used for the Yushu earthquake rescue was simpler. It contained only one step: directly transporting patients from the disaster areas to rear hospitals. Severely injured patients were transported to 54 general, specialized, and traditional Chinese hospitals in seven cities (Xi'ning, Hainan district, Golmud, Lanzhou, Xi'an, Chengdu, Qamdo) and five provinces.

Evacuation Methods

Ground and aerial transport vehicles were used for medical evacuation during the Wenchuan earthquake rescue. The transportation department of the army and those overseeing civilian aviation, railways, and highways were involved in patients' medical evacuation, and they provided ambulances, helicopters, medical trains, etc. Airplanes and trains were the main vehicles that were used for trans-provincial evacuation. Aeromedical evacuation rescued 97.7 % of the severely injured in Wenchuan, Mao county, and Li county.

Yushu is located on a plateau, and it was difficult for ground transportation to play a major role in evacuation. Except for the first group of patients that was transported by bus after the earthquake to Xining, only a handful of patients were transported by ambulance or private cars to HaiNaZhou, Tibet, and other adjacent regions, and the vast majority of patients were transported by air. The aircraft used in the AE mission included IL-76 transport aircrafts from the Air Force, Airbus A-319s from civil aviation, and MI-17 helicopters from Army aviation. From April 15 to May 5, there were a total of 152 flights, of which 95 were by Airbus 124 A319, 53 by IL-76, and 5 by MI-17 helicopter. In addition, on April 24, 174 patients were transported again by train from Xining, Qinghai province, to Xi'an and Lanzhou for follow-up treatment (Liu et al. 2013).

Treatment in Echelon

In this section, emergency medical relief will be presented as a "three-stage" treatment. During the first 72 h after an earthquake, first aid plays a key role. From 72 h to 2 weeks after an earthquake, emergency treatment and early treatment (damage control treatment) are the main treatment methods. Two weeks after an earthquake, patients begin to receive specialist treatment (deterministic treatment). After the Wenchuan earthquake, seriously wounded people were treated in large comprehensive hospitals located outside of the disaster areas according to the principle of concentrated treatment. The number of deaths accounted for 2.98 % of the total number of people who were hospitalized.

The rescue strategy for Yushu earthquake relief was more coherent than other strategies that had been constructed for previous earthquakes. Transportation of the wounded, specialist treatment, and rehabilitation guidance were realized in the early stage. Seven days after the earthquake, rehabilitation experts began to guide patients toward receiving rehabilitation treatment so as to guarantee a low death rate and disability rate. During the Yushu earthquake relief process, all of the seriously injured were evacuated for treatment. The number of deaths accounted for only 0.10 % of the total number of people hospitalized.

4.1.2.2 The Current Situation (Wenchuan and Yushu)

Early Evacuation and Simple Evacuation Echelon Meet the Demand of Patients' Treatment Needs

The traditional "three-step" program was used for Wenchuan medical evacuation. Practice showed that the traditional medical evacuation system, which suited military operation, seemed to require too much hierarchy and had the possibility of leading to low emergency efficiency in disaster rescue. Foreign disaster medical rescue experience showed that patients' survival rate and their prognosis could be improved by shortening the time it took for them to be sent from the site of injury to a site of medical treatment. Studying the results of the Pakistan earthquake and Hurricane Katrina indicated that rehabilitation experts should begin to guide patients in the early stage (Akbari et al. 2004; Urbina and Wolshon 2003). In the Yushu earthquake rescue, the evacuation echelon was simplified to one step. Patients were directly sent from the disaster areas to rear hospitals where they could enjoy specialist treatment. This simplification ensured the timeliness of specialized treatment, greatly shortened the time from first aid to hospitalization, guaranteed early individualized treatment and rehabilitation, and reduced the morbidity of quake victims.

Standardization Degree of Patients' Triage Is Not Enough

During the Wenchuan earthquake rescue, some severely injured people were not processed in a timely and correct fashion due to the lack of professional triage personnel. Some lightly injured people preferred evacuation. According to statistics about the Wenchuan earthquake, the proportion of lightly injured people was as high as 32 % of the total patients evacuated by helicopter (Zhang et al. 2011). This caused a great waste of scarce resources such as medical transport capacity. In the Yushu earthquake rescue, people who were transferred to the superior, specialized subject hospital accounted for 1/3 of the 257 patients transported twice to another hospital. As a result of unqualified triage at the disaster areas, the excessive triage or insufficient triage of patients abounded. In earthquake relief, therefore, professional triage personnel should be sent to the disaster areas, relatively standardized triage criteria should be established, the waste of rescue resources should be reduced, and the delay of patients' treatment time should be avoided (Nie et al. 2011; Xiang et al. 2009).

Evaluation of the Holding Ability of Rear Hospitals

After the Wenchuan earthquake, about 10,452 (22 %) of the patients were admitted to hospitals within 72 h, and the number of hospitalized patients in a week accounted for 62.8–74.75 % of the total. After the Yushu earthquake, nearly 1,434 severely injured patients were evacuated within 72 h, and more than 90 % of patients were admitted to a hospital in the first week (Kang et al. 2012). In addition, comprehensive factors such as the state of an illness and subsequent placement often led to a long hospitalized time, which increased the pressure on rear hospitals. After the Yushu earthquake on April 24, 169 patients were transported again from Xining, Qinghai province, to Xi'an and Lanzhou. The reason given for the transfer was "to alleviate the workload of Xining City's rear hospital," indicating that evaluating whether the occupancy load could meet the demand of the number of hospitalized patients while selecting a rear hospital was necessary.

Aeromedical Evacuation Played an Important Role, but the Airplanes Were Not Qualified for Safety Evacuation

Because of their high speed and lack of restriction by road conditions, aircraft have been frequently used in post-disaster rescue operations for the evacuation of casualties since the 1980s. Because we do not have any special medical aircraft, the airplanes that participated in the Wenchuan and Yushu earthquake medical evacuations were military transport aircraft, civil passenger planes, and military helicopters. They were not specially designed or modified for medical evacuation, so they often lacked medical equipment. This was a hidden danger for patients' security.

4.1.3 Objective and Significance

4.1.3.1 Purpose of Research

Guided by the research concept of evidence-informed decision making, we (a) analyzed the orientation, characteristics, mechanisms, and principles of earthquake medical evacuation; (b) revealed the subject's behavior characteristics and the law of the system evolution of earthquake medical evacuation systems; (c) built a logical model and an SD model of an earthquake medical evacuation system; (d) via a simulation and policy intervention experiment, discovered the root of the system structure barriers and function mechanism; and (e) put forward policy suggestions to help solve the structural problems of evacuation systems. Our research results can be helpful to earthquake relief emergency medical rescue decision making and provide quantitative research for earthquake medical evacuation planning.

4.1.3.2 Research Significance

In this study, we first built a system dynamics model of an earthquake medical evacuation system, which can provide an experimental platform for policy intervention study and evidence for scientific decision making. This model extends complex system science and the theory of complex adaptive methods in the emergency medical rescue research area, and it could provide methods to scientific decision and quantitative research for earthquake medical evacuation.

4.2 Data Resources Used in the Earthquake Medical Evacuation Model

4.2.1 Utilization of the Current Data Resources

1. Basic Information About All Previous Earthquakes, Both Local and Nonlocal, Was Mainly Retrieved from the Internet
2. More than 100 copies of overseas earthquake medical evacuation literature were retrieved by databases including Medline, Pubmed, Proquest, ELSEVIER, THTF, and CQVIP.
3. More than 100 copies of documents, reports, and statistics about the Yushu earthquake emergency medical rescue operation were retrieved from the National Ministry of Health (Chart 4.1).

Time	Place	Data collection
April 2010	Yushu, Qinghai	Interviewed commanders of front-line medical disaster relief agencies; Expert interviews
August 2010	Beijing	Collection of arrangement of files from the Ministry of Health, Data analysis; Expert interviews
December 2010	Qinghai	Collection and arrangement of files from Qinghai Province Health Department; Survey of regional support forces; Survey of disaster rescue forces; Survey of the medical evacuation of casualties; Expert interviews and discussion forum
February 2011	Sichuan, Gansu, Shanxi, Xizang	Survey of rear hospital treatment; Survey of strategic support force

Chart 4.1 Schedule of the on-site survey of the Yushu earthquake emergency medical rescue

4. More than 50 copies of public documents related to the use of troops in the Yushu earthquake relief emergency medical rescue were retrieved. More than 80 copies of earthquake relief brief reports were retrieved from a military medical university.
5. Domestic disaster medical rescue research results that were published in recent years were also retrieved.

4.2.2 Data Sources from Field Surveys

4.2.2.1 On-Site Survey of the Wenchuan Earthquake Relief Emergency Medical Rescue Operation

Data and Respondents

Beginning on June 13, 2008, our research group conducted a 10-day on-site investigation in the Wenchuan earthquake disaster areas. The condition of the sick and wounded in the cities of Mianyang, Mianzhu, Dujiangyan, and Pengzhou; the counties of Beichuan, Anxian, and Maoxian; and the town of Yingxiu was investigated. Medical rescue headquarters at all levels, including the medical team commander's headquarters, each general's headquarters, AOR headquarters, the army-civilian joint command headquarters, and the National Health Ministry working group, were investigated. Surveys were given to all kinds of medical rescue teams, including strategic support powers, the rescue squads and local medical personnel sent by various provinces and cities, and army medical aid. All kinds of medical rescue teams, including strategic support medical forces, rescue detachments from many provinces and cities, local medical personnel, and military medical rescue forces, were surveyed. The types of teams that we surveyed included medical teams, epidemic prevention teams, psychological aid teams, seven field hospitals (including two field shelter hospitals), rear hospitals, and local and nationwide medical institutions.

Survey Methods

We mainly used interviews, small meetings, and focus group interviews in our investigation, and an interview outline was set for every interview. More than 50 first-line medical experts and medical rescue leaders from all levels were interviewed. More than ten small conferences at rear hospitals were held with medical rescue personnel from all levels and various medical rescue teams. Focus group interviews on a given research topic were held three times. Interview results were recorded in the form of texts and audio recordings. The data was organized after the research. Medical rescue experts were given the option to have a brainstorming session during the forum. In the interviews, researchers and respondents could discuss the problems of medical rescue and put forward solutions to them.

Research Content

The research content of this project was defined by the respondents. Research content for the rescue institutions included the number and source of the sick and wounded, the triage standard, the system of and vehicles for medical evacuation, and the personnel allocation for medical evacuation. Research content for the medical rescue command institutes included command system, institution rank, coordination mechanism, and use of medical forces.

Quality Control

In the interview investigation, an interview outline was drawn up in advance according to previous research, and data summary was conducted on the same day. All team members were responsible for recording the interview process.

4.2.2.2 On-Site Survey of the Yushu Earthquake Relief Emergency Medical Rescue Operation

Data and Respondents

Investigation of the Yushu earthquake relief efforts was conducted in four stages.

First, our research group conducted a 4-day on-site investigation of the Yushu earthquake disaster areas beginning in April 2008, and we collected a large number of medical rescue related documents from an earthquake relief area command.

Second, our research group conducted a 5-day Yushu earthquake emergency medical rescue data collection and assessment at the National Health Ministry (Beijing) in October 2010. This data included: (1) related files of the National Health Ministry,; (2) duty information of the National Health Ministry,; (3) general information about the epidemic prevention personnel and vehicles that were dispatched to the Yushu earthquake disaster areas of Qinghai province,; (4) reported information statistical tables of the Health Ministry,; (5) statistics from the physical distribution working group,; (6) meeting minutes of the Health Ministry and medical emergency leading group of Yushu earthquake of Qinghai province,; (7) an information sheet about post-disaster reconstruction,; and (8) report forms for physical distribution.

Third, our research group conducted a 1-week retrospective investigation in Xi'ning city of Qinghai province in December 2010. Respondents included medical rescue institutions, health administrative departments, and medical rescue personnel. The surveyed health administrative institutions included the Qinghai province emergency office of the health department, the medical administration bureau, and the health bureau of Yushu prefecture. More than ten medical services institution were surveyed, including People's Hospital of Qinghai Province and Affiliated Hospital of Qinghai University.

Fourth, our research group conducted a supplementary survey in the Sichuan, Shaanxi, and Gansu provinces and the Tibet Autonomous Region from January to February 2011. The survey mainly investigated the hospitals to which the evacuated sick and wounded were admitted.

Survey Methods

Our investigation mainly used interviews, small meetings, and focus group interviews. Our interview of experts included three face-to-face interviews with leaders from the Qinghai province health department and Yushu prefecture. More than 40 people, including health administrative personnel, medical personnel, and health supervision personnel, were invited to three small discussions. Interview results were recorded in the form of texts and audio recordings. Organization of data was conducted after the research. A questionnaire survey was mainly given to the medical personnel who took part in earthquake emergency medical relief, including more than 300 medical personnel from Qinghai province and more than 120 personnel from Yushu County. A supplementary survey was mainly conducted through making phone calls and asking people to fill in forms on an online questionnaire that delegated answers to the Health Departments of the Shan'xi, Gansu, and Tibet provinces. All the results were sent back to the research group via email or mail.

Research Content

1. Occurrence of the sick and wounded
2. The structure of the emergency medical rescue command at the national, provincial, and disaster area levels
3. The allocation and admission of emergency medical forces to local and rear hospitals
4. The interviews held with more than 60 medical experts and principals associated with the emergency medical rescue at all levels
5. The more than 10 symposia held with the injured who were admitted to hospitals, medical rescue personnel at all levels, and various rescue squads
6. 378 copies of questionnaires that were given out to support medical team members, medical workers in the air transfer station, and local rescue team members
7. More than 500 copies of related documents and report forms.

Quality Control

The interviews provided a thorough venue for detailed data collection. Each interview question was discussed according to a detailed interview outline. The team members listened to the views and opinions of the respondents and meeting personnel, and they were responsible for keeping the records and systemizing them.

Before the questionnaire survey was administered, a research group member elaborated the significance of the research to the participants and explained the key subjects item by item in order to guarantee the quality of completed questionnaires. In Yushu county, local bureau of health personnel helped explain the content of the local medical personnel questionnaire survey item by item, and issues related to language differences were avoided.

4.2.3 Collection of Literature

More than 140 articles were published from 2002 to 2012 related to earthquake relief rescue evacuation, and essays focusing on rescue simulation and modeling were selected from sources such as Chinese Journal of Evidence-Based Medicine, Chinese Critical Care Medicine, Journal of Trauma Surgery, Hospitals Administration Journal of Chinese PLA, China Journal of Emergency Resuscitation and Disaster Medicine, Emergency Medical Journal, and Journal of Trauma by manual retrieval from databases such as Medline, ProQuest, PubMed, and Chinese Biomedical Literature Database.

4.3 Construction of the Earthquake Medical Evacuation Model

4.3.1 Concept Model of the Earthquake Medical Evacuation

In the construction of a conceptual model of earthquake relief medical evacuation system (MES), three subjects were highlighted: the headquarters, the medical evacuation organizations at all levels (the suppliers), and the sick and wounded (the buyers).

The sick and wounded flowed independently into the system on the basis of injuries and systematic rules. Medical evacuation organizations at all levels (the suppliers) adjusted the structure of internal resources allocation according to the supply of medical evacuation resources. The three subjects of the supplier (the on-site treatment system, evacuation system, and the rear hospital system) interacted with each other through stock resource adjustment and incremental resources allocation behavior. The headquarters improved the efficiency of the system as a whole by executing macro command decisions and promoting good coordination between the systems, which helped maintain high efficiency and improve the utilization rate of resources. Interaction among all subjects constituted a driving force for the structural evolution of earthquake relief MES.

The evolution of the supplier system structure, the subjects' behavior, and the coordination mechanism of the earthquake relief MES subsystem were the foci of this modeling research.

4.3.2 *Logic Model of Earthquake Medical Evacuation*

The internal environment of earthquake relief MES and its complex interrelations with seismic situations, natural geography, and social environments are interconnected, interdependent, and interactional. This research mainly focused on the behavior mechanism of MES in an earthquake rescue and management system. The first-line treatment system, evacuation system, and rear hospital system were constructed, respectively. The earthquake relief MES logical model is constructed by the decomposition and synthesis of the subjects' body behavior analysis and main loop analysis (Fig. 4.1).

4.3.3 *SD Model of Earthquake Medical Evacuation*

4.3.3.1 Assumptions of Earthquake Relief MES Modeling

The evolutionary process of the earthquake relief MES structure is complex, dynamic, and continuous, and it is difficult to use the system dynamics of complex systems to simulate the whole process of this complex system dynamic evolution.

Therefore, in the process of earthquake relief MES modeling, this research assumed that the initial structure would remain static. In other words, we assumed that the structural elements of the system would remain unchanged within a certain time while the system structure would vary according to the possession of its own resources. The evolution of the system structure was judged by observing the change of the structure index after a stable system structure was achieved.

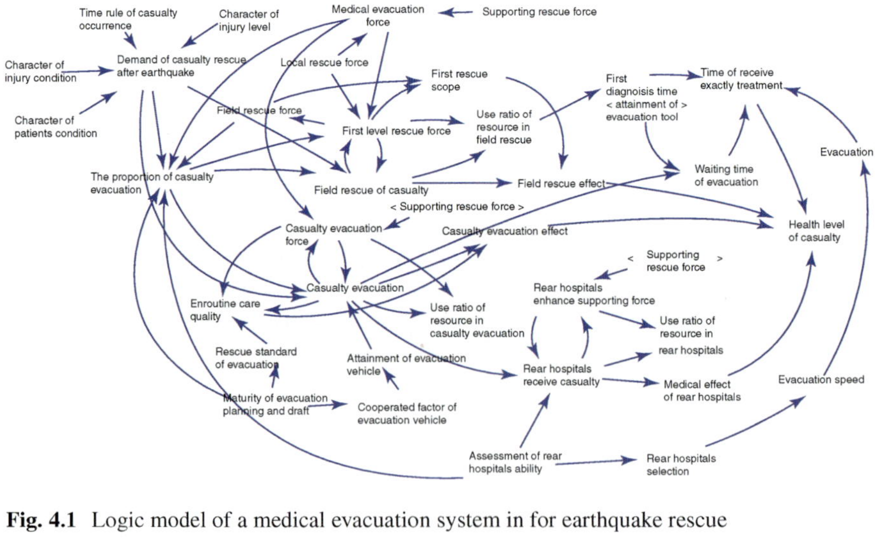

Fig. 4.1 Logic model of a medical evacuation system in for earthquake rescue

For the purposes of scientific disaster relief, the logical framework of this system structure should contain structures for emergency medical rescue resources allocation and organization. It would then be able to provide a basis for discussions about macro and micro emergency medical aid decision making that will match the system structure and the external environment. The treatment requirements of the sick and wounded and resource allocation efficiency should be also taken into consideration in order to maximize the total benefit of earthquake relief.

Disaster relief medical evacuation consists of the emergency medical rescue operations that follow great earthquake disasters. The abruptness and destructiveness of earthquakes require an emergency medical rescue system that can rapidly respond and is of high quality. Velocity and quality are important measures for measuring the efficiency of disaster relief emergency medical rescue. Efficiency and effectiveness are important indices for evaluating earthquake relief emergency medical rescue operations. In this study, the goal of earthquake relief MES is assumed to improve the treatment effectiveness of medical evacuation in earthquake relief medical rescue operations, shorten the evacuation time, and optimize the allocation of resources in order to improve the effect and efficiency of MES in earthquake relief to the maximum.

The following were selected as our main observation indices: completion rate of the evacuation, effective cure rate, medical resources utilization, and medical resource low efficiency loss in disaster areas. To better observe the MES in earthquake relief operation, the daily patients evacuated and the change of the system resource structure were selected as auxiliary observation indices.

Based on the main causation analysis of the system, main policy intervention indices of the earthquake relief commander to MES included the following: evacuation decision making, supporting medical resources allocation, adjusting time of resources, medical evacuation plan, and emergency management. These indices were reflected in the following ways: the initial value of the evacuation decision (evacuation time, evacuation ratio, etc.), status of medical forces adjustment, and organization and command.

4.3.3.2 Main Variables and Functions of the Earthquake Relief MES Models

Parameter estimation, system dynamics, econometrics, expert consultation, brainstorming, and field investigation were used synthetically to determine the main variables. Different methods were used according to the different types of parameters in order to determine the mathematical function relation of each equation.

Flow Variables

Flow variables included the accumulated number of the wounded, the accumulated number of the wounded who were cured, the accumulated number of patients, the accumulated number of cured patients, the number of patients taken in daily, the number of evacuated patients, supporting medical forces, the accumulated number of supporting medical forces that retreated, the medical evacuation decision making, the medical evacuation plan, the organization and command, and the medical demand judgment.

Flow Rate Variables

Flow rate variables included the daily number of people who had been wounded, the daily number of sick and wounded people that were evacuated, the daily number of wounded people who were cured, the daily number of added patients, the daily number of cured patients, and the daily number of added inpatients. Other important variables included the following: information rate, information acquisition, project completion, decision making, and implementation.

Auxiliary Variables

Auxiliary variables included the average length of stay for patients with mild symptoms, the average length of treatment for patients who stayed for observation, the average length of stay for surgery patients, and the standard treatment rate.

Initial Variables

Initial variables included the start time of the evacuation, the evacuation ratio, and the total number of medical teams, local medical forces, standard judgment, standard organization, and standard decision making.

Observation Variables

Observation variables included the completion rate of effective treatment, the utilization of medical resources in disaster areas, and the low efficiency loss of medical resources in disaster areas.

Smooth Function

Smooth function serves as an information delay. Smooth function is divided into first-order smooth and third-order smooth, and it is akin to an organizing implementation rate.

Delay Function

A delay that happens in a logistics line is called a logistical delay. A delay is a phenomenon in which a variable manifests after the time that it is supposed to. For example, it will take some time for supporting medical forces to prepare in order to depart for disaster areas. After people become sick or are wounded, it will also take some time for them to enter the medical evacuation system and triage, where they can then be reckoned in the number of the sick and wounded. The above two variables are a first-order logistical index delay function.

Logical Functions

Logical functions included MAX, MIN, and IF THEN ELSE. In this research, IF THEN ELSE and MIN were primarily used. The IF THEN ELSE logical function included the join and retreat of the first-line supporting forces.

Table Function

Table function was set on the base of analysis of on-site research data, initial identification of the extremum, and the median of those variables, and it sets the happening ratio of daily patients and the evacuation ratio by expert consultation so as to clarify their changing trend.

Initial Value

Initial values were set by the Yushu earthquake relief memorabilia of the National Ministry of Health, daily briefing and related statements, and the tactical and technical index found in the "Military Health Service Science," which were combined with expert consultations, interviews, and on-site research data.

4.4 Simulation and Intervention of the Earthquake Medical Evacuation Model

4.4.1 Systemic Simulation

The time length of the dynamic simulation model is 30 days, and the step size is 1 day as follows:

4.4.1.1 Simulation of the Sick and Wounded Accumulation

Evacuation work was carried out steadily on the given evacuating ratio after orders were received from the earthquake relief general headquarters. The evacuation task was completed in 1 week (Fig. 4.2).

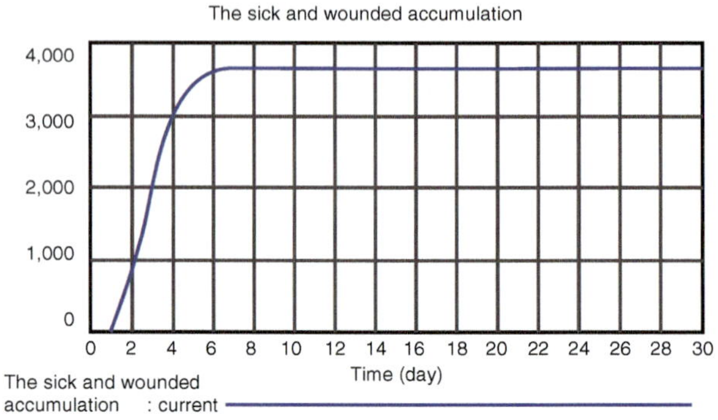

Fig. 4.2 Simulation of the sick and wounded accumulation

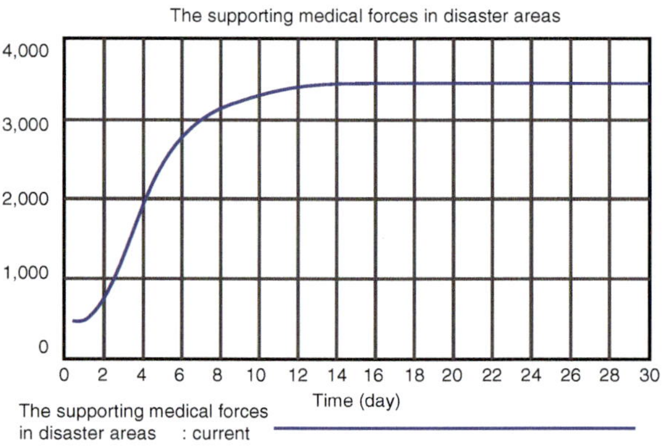

Fig. 4.3 Simulation of the supporting medical forces in disaster areas

4.4.1.2 Simulation of the Medical Evacuation Resources

Simulation of the Medical Forces in Disaster Areas

It took some time to establish a national earthquake relief headquarters that could send parties to disaster areas, draw supporting medical forces to disaster areas, and deliver medical services.

After a quick supporting forces transfer, preparation, and mobility, the medical forces in disaster areas increased gradually and peaked on the 8th or 9th day (Figs. 4.3 and 4.4).

The supporting medical forces that arrived in the disaster areas within 72 h were limited. Most supporting medical forces (including field shelter hospitals) arrived between the 3rd and 7th days. This may be related to transfer velocity, preparation time, and mobility.

The critical period of medical rescue is 24 h after an earthquake, 8 h is a critical period for life saving, and specialists best exert their function within 72 h. Therefore, low resource allocation efficiency for the supporting medical forces in disaster areas within 72 h of an earthquake is the main obstacle of resource structures.

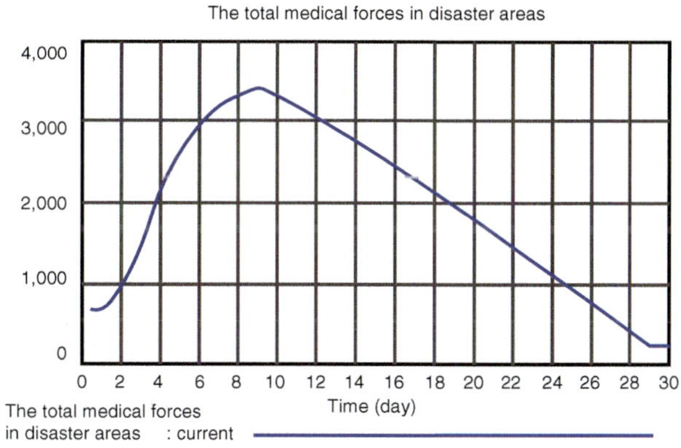

Fig. 4.4 Simulation of the total medical forces in disaster areas

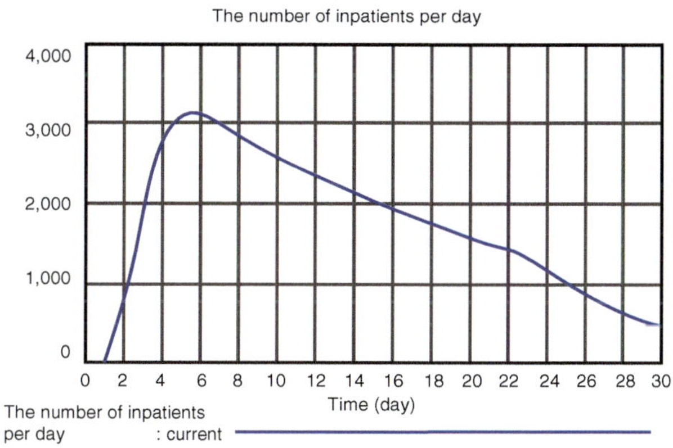

Fig. 4.5 Simulation of the inpatients in rear hospitals

On the 8th day of the earthquake, health and epidemic prevention groups from the earthquake relief headquarters began to organize the drawback of support medical forces. The above figure shows that medical forces in the disaster areas tapered off starting around the 9th day after the earthquake. All emergency medical teams but two military field shelter hospitals retreated on the 30th day after the earthquake.

Simulation of the Inpatients in Rear Hospitals

The number of inpatients in rear hospitals rose as the sick and wounded evacuated, peaked between the 5th and 7th days after the earthquake, and then dropped slowly. More than 50 % of inpatients were still in hospitals for treatments even 3 weeks after the earthquake. The lasting high medical demand was probably related to traumatic conditions, illness conditions, and follow-up arrangements (Fig. 4.5).

4.4.1.3 Simulation of the Medical Evacuation Effect

The first evacuation of the sick and wounded was completed in 1 week.

The effective cure rate rose gradually with the development of the earthquake emergency medical rescue, and all disaster areas were covered on the 9th day. Medical forces in disaster areas reached a saturation point, and the effective cure rate rose to 100 % (Fig. 4.6).

The number of medical forces continued to increase after the earthquake, and they met the demands for field treatment on the 5th day while the medical forces in the disaster areas reached a saturation point and attained an effective cure rate of 100 % (Fig. 4.7). However, the number of medical forces still increased. Following the 5th day after the quake, the medical forces were greater than the demand for resources, which increased the low efficiency of power loss due to the waste of resources. The adjustment of the medical forces started on the 8th day; meanwhile, supporting medical forces began to leave. Low efficiency of power loss decreased gradually and reached the zero point on the 30th day (Fig. 4.8).

4.4.2 *Intervention*

4.4.2.1 Policy Group Selecting

To observe the impact of system parameters on system behavior and results, four groups of intervention experiments were designed to observe the simulation results received by adjusting the initial value of the evacuation decision, adjusting the time of

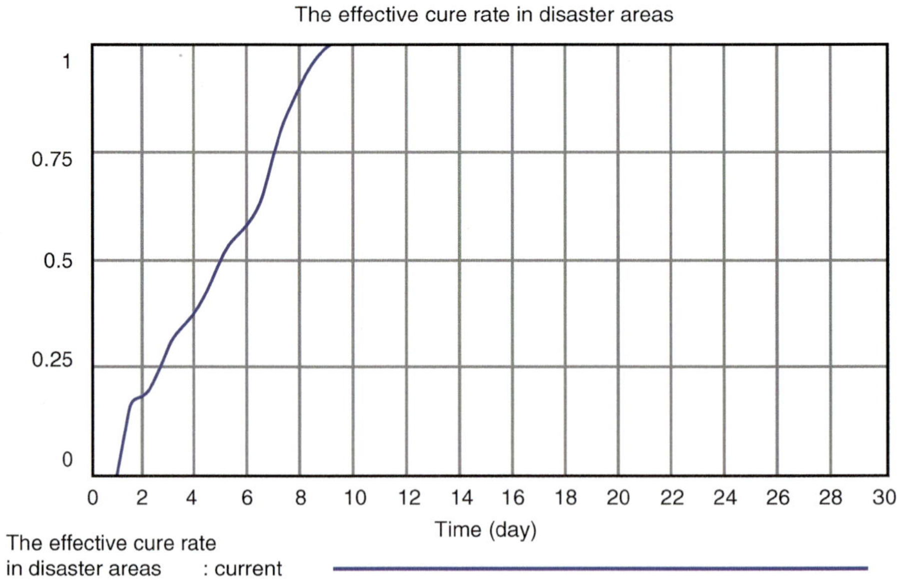

Fig. 4.6 Simulation of the effective cure rate in disaster areas

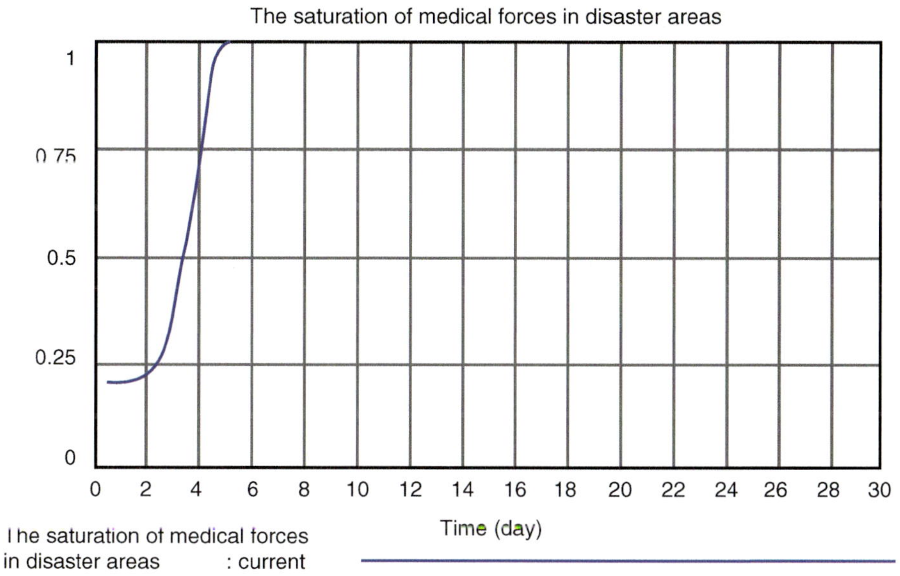

Fig. 4.7 Simulation of how medical forces saturation in disaster areas

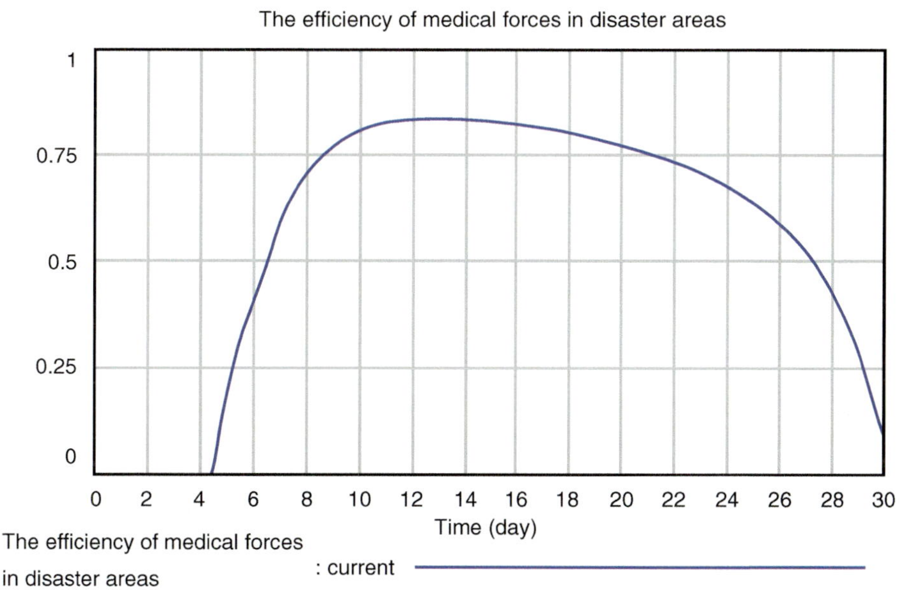

Fig. 4.8 Simulation of the efficiency of medical forces in disaster areas

the organization command initial value to observe the patients in the earthquake relief MES treatment efficiency, and changing the efficiency of medical forces allocation.

Adjusting the Initial Value of the Evacuation Decision

We observed the start time variation and ratio (triage index) of evacuation to see whether an advanced evacuation time, a higher effective treatment rate, and a different value of treatment needs in the rear hospitals would be achieved.

Adjustment of the Timing of Regulating the Medical Forces in Disaster Areas

We observed the moving up or delay of medical forces in disaster areas to see what would happen to the saturability and low efficiency of power loss of the medical forces and whether a higher medical resource allocation efficiency would be achieved.

Adjusting the Initial Value of the Organization and Command Subsystem

We observed and adjusted the preparation status of medical need; evacuation plan; and evacuation decision making, organization, and commanding to see how the complete time and medical forces allocation efficiency would change.

4.4.2.2 Adjustment of the Initial Value of the Evacuation Decision

Adjustment of the Starting Time of the Evacuation

To observe the influence of the evacuation starting time on the treatment efficiency, three groups of intervention experiments were designed to conduct the model simulation (Fig. 4.9a, b).

Current: Evacuating the sick and wounded on the 1st day of the earthquake
Test 1: Evacuating the sick and wounded on the 3rd day of the earthquake
Test 2: Evacuating the sick and wounded on the 10th day of the earthquake

The results of the intervention experiments showed that the completion of evacuation would be earlier while the effective treatment rate would be higher. Effective treatment rate: Current>Test 1>Test2, which may be related to how the earlier evacuation of severely wounded relieved the conflict between rescue demand and limited medical forces in the disaster areas. In Yushu earthquake relief, the principle of early evacuation and evacuating all severely wounded, along with evacuation on the 1st day, helped the inpatient casualty rate stay at 0.1 % (Fig. 4.9a, b).

Jiegu, the town where the epicenter of the Yushu earthquake was located, is linked to the outside world by National Highway 214 and Batang airport. Located

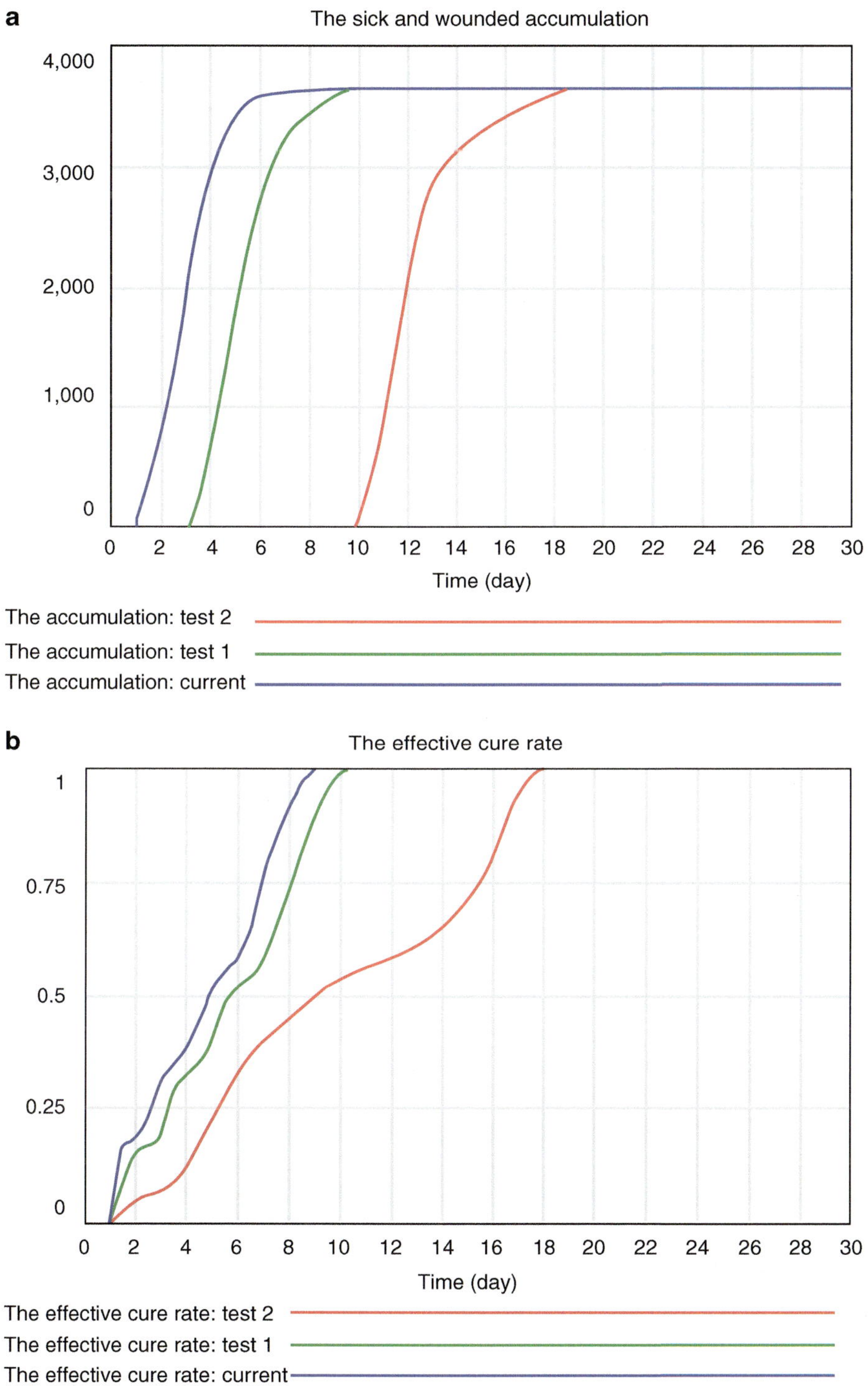

Fig. 4.9 (**a**) Simulation of the effective cure rate in disaster areas (variation of the sick and wounded accumulation). (**b**) Simulation of the effective cure rate in disaster areas (variation of the effective cure rate)

about 18 km south of Jiegu, the Batang airport has the fourth highest altitude (at 3905 m) of an airport in China, and it was put into use on August 1, 2009. The earthquake did not cause serious damage to the airport, and planes could take off and land on the day of the earthquake, which provided an excellent traffic condition for evacuating the sick and wounded. Therefore, in a proper traffic condition and earthquake situation, early evacuation of the sick and wounded could not only shorten the time it takes for them to receive specialist treatments, but it could also reduce the treatment demand of severely injured people in disaster areas and improve the effective treatment rate.

Adjusting the Initial Value of the Evacuation Ratio

To observe the influence of the evacuation ratio on evacuation and treatment efficiency, three groups of intervention experiments were designed to conduct the model simulation.

Current: Evacuating initial ratio is set at 0.3
Test 1: Evacuating initial ratio is set at 0.01
Test 2: Evacuating initial ratio is set at 0.8

The evacuation ratio is usually predicted by the disaster relief medical rescue headquarters on the basis of the earthquake situation, the number of casualties, and the capacity of available vehicles. Intervention results showed that under the condition of a certain amount of evacuation vehicles, a rising evacuating ratio would result in a prolonged time for completing evacuations. However, reducing the evacuation ratio would not shorten the evacuation time significantly (Fig. 4.10a, b). This is because evacuation is decided by how the situation of patients unfolds every day. The evacuation completing time in Test 1 and Current shows no significant difference, which shows that evacuation vehicles' capacity met the requirements of evacuation need and basically accorded with the time sequence of sick and wounded people in Current. The effective treatment rate in disaster areas was reduced, and the utilization of evacuation vehicles was insufficient in Test 1. In Test 2, the evacuation ratio was too large and surpassed the capacity of evacuating vehicles, which delayed the complete time of evacuation and did not increase the rate of effective treatment. Figure 4.10c shows that a proper evacuation ratio might reduce evacuation time and guarantee a high effective treatment rate.

For the demands of the rear hospitals, the evacuation ratio change did not affect daily changes in the rate of hospitalized patients. Hospitalized patients were increasing daily and declined gradually after the peak in three situations. Figure 4.10d shows that after the number of inpatients peaked in rear hospitals, the inpatient demand peaked for 2–4 weeks. Many patients still stayed in hospitals, which suggested that rear hospitals should consider the balance between the long-term treatment demand of the inpatients and daily medical services. After the Yushu earthquake, some patients in Xining were transferred again to Lanzhou of Gansu and Xi'an of Shaanxi to complete their follow-up rehabilitation in order to alleviate

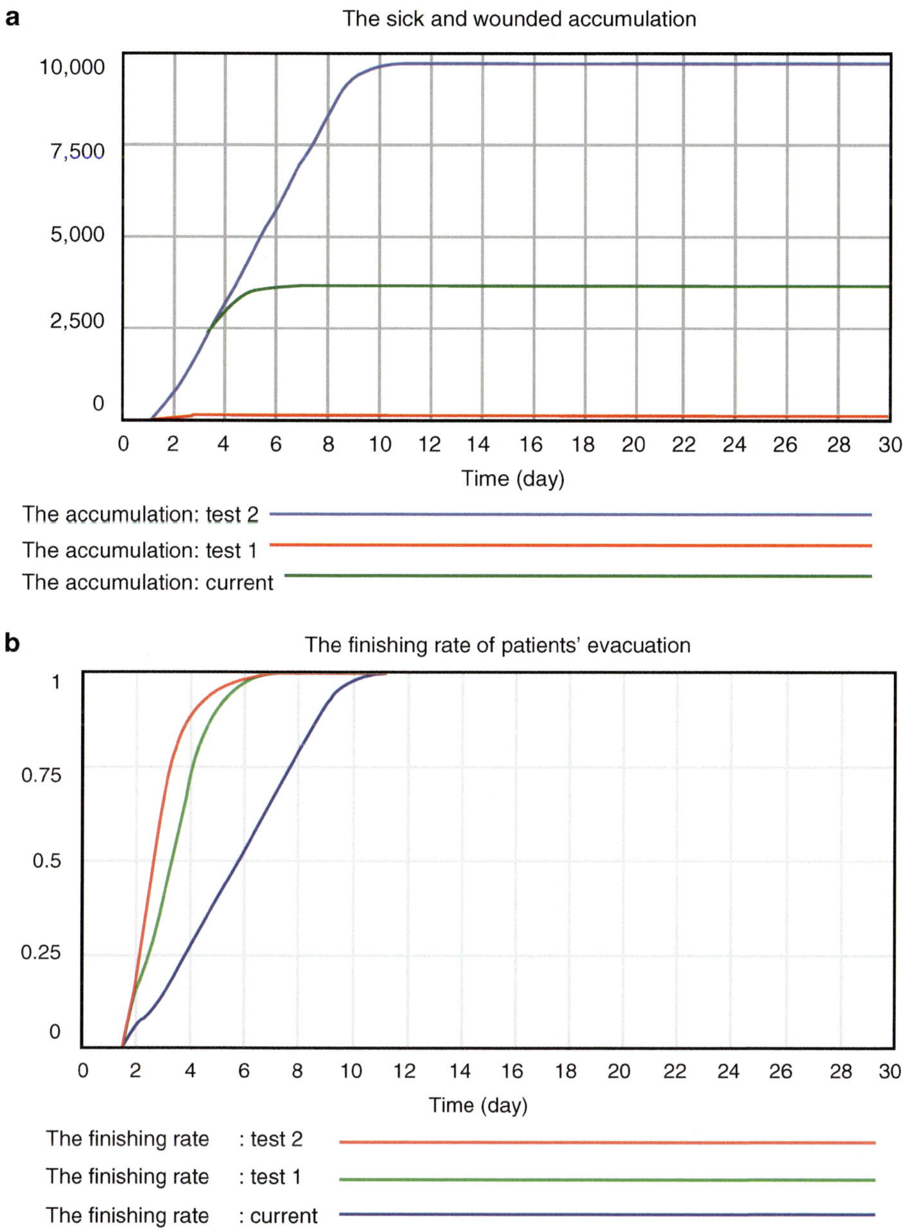

Fig. 4.10 (**a**) Simulation of the effective cure rate in disaster areas (variation of the sick and wounded accumulation). (**b**) Simulation of the effective cure rate in disaster areas (variation of the finishing rate of patients' evacuation). (**c**) Simulation of the effective cure rate in disaster areas (variation of the effective cure rate). (**d**) Simulation of the effective cure rate in disaster areas (variation in the number of inpatients)

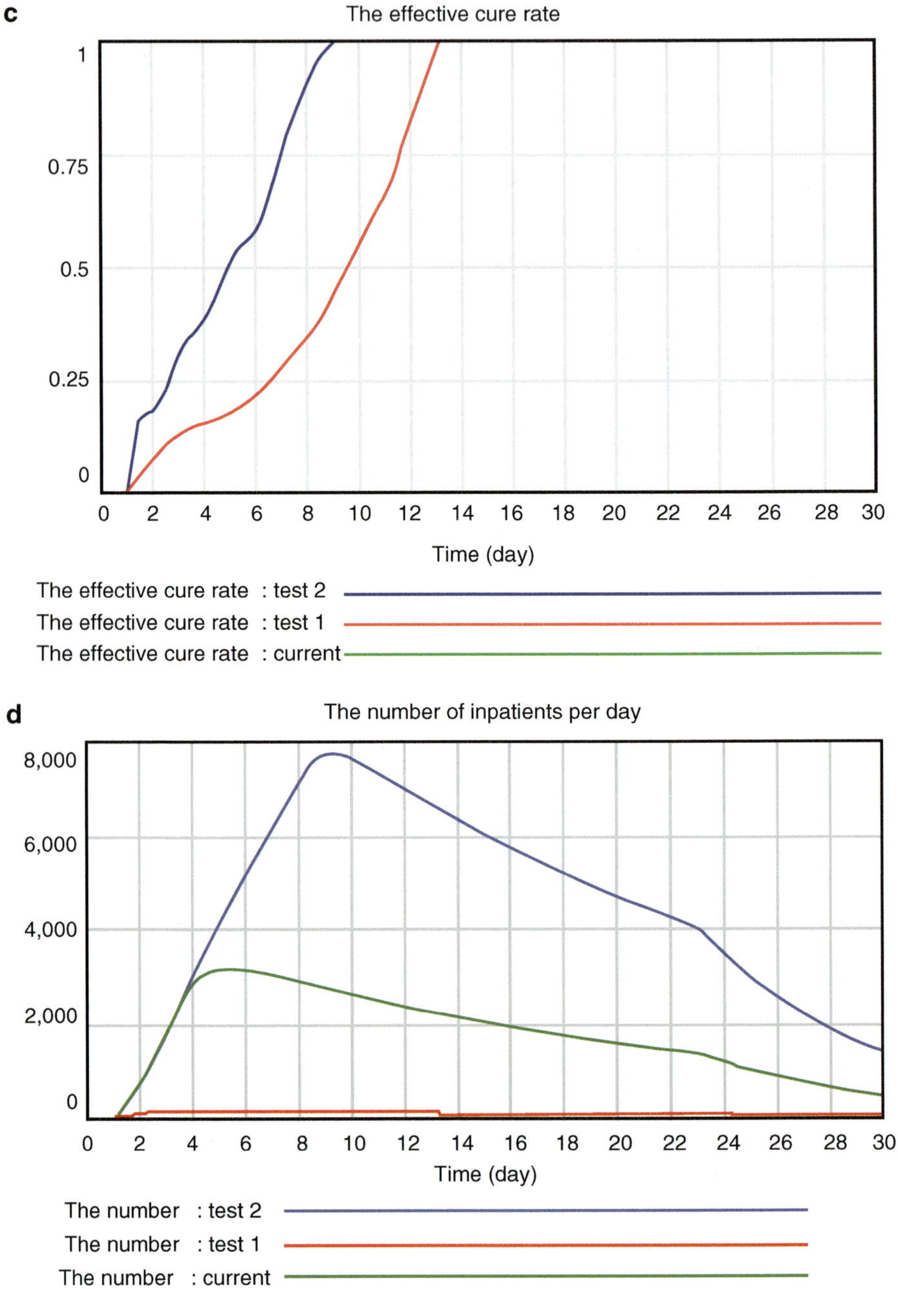

Fig. 4.10 (continued)

the pressure on the Xining rear hospital. Having to transfer patients more than once means that rear hospitals were insufficiently prepared for the peaking of treatment demand.

The evacuation ratio is an important index for triage treatment. Proper evacuation standards have a positive role to play in relieving disaster treatment pressure and improving the use of evacuation vehicles and rear hospital resources. Because the evacuation ratio is affected by the geography, traffic conditions, and seismic conditions found in the disaster areas and the expected number of sick and wounded, the disaster relief medical rescue headquarters should adjust the evacuation ratio dynamically according to information updates in order to guarantee the effectiveness of evacuations and resource allocation.

Adjusting the Time of Medical Forces in Disaster Areas

To observe the influence of the timely adjustment of medical forces in disaster areas on treatment efficiency, three groups of intervention experiments were designed to conduct the model simulation.

Current: Adjusting the medical forces in disaster areas after the 7th day
Test 1: Adjusting the medical forces in disaster areas after the 3rd day
Test 2: Adjusting the medical forces in disaster areas after the 15th day

Intervention results showed that adjusting the time that disaster medical forces stayed in disaster areas had no effect on the saturation of medical forces, but there was an obvious impact on the efficiency of disaster medical forces. The low efficiency losses of the medical forces were Test 1>Current>Test 2 (Fig. 4.11a, b). As the disaster medical forces adjusted in advance, the low efficiency of disaster medical forces loss decreased significantly and medical forces allocation efficiency improved.

In the two on-site investigations we conducted, medical rescue commanders and team members agreed that specialized medical personnel play a key role within 72 h after the quake and can be withdrawn after 72 h. Medical forces should make their rounds as early as possible. Specialists could take turns for supplementing them. Medical forces began to retreat on the 9th day after the Yushu earthquake. All the supporting forces from other provinces, except military field shelter hospitals, retreated on the 17th day after the earthquake. On the 30th day, regional supporting forces retreated as well.

However, the results of intervention showed that the low situation of medical forces in disaster areas within 72 h did not improve along with the adjustment time, which suggests that the saturation of medical forces may be related to the lagging allocation of supporting forces compared with the drawing, the commanding and decision-making efficiency, and the mobility of medical forces. We will continue to discuss the next experiments.

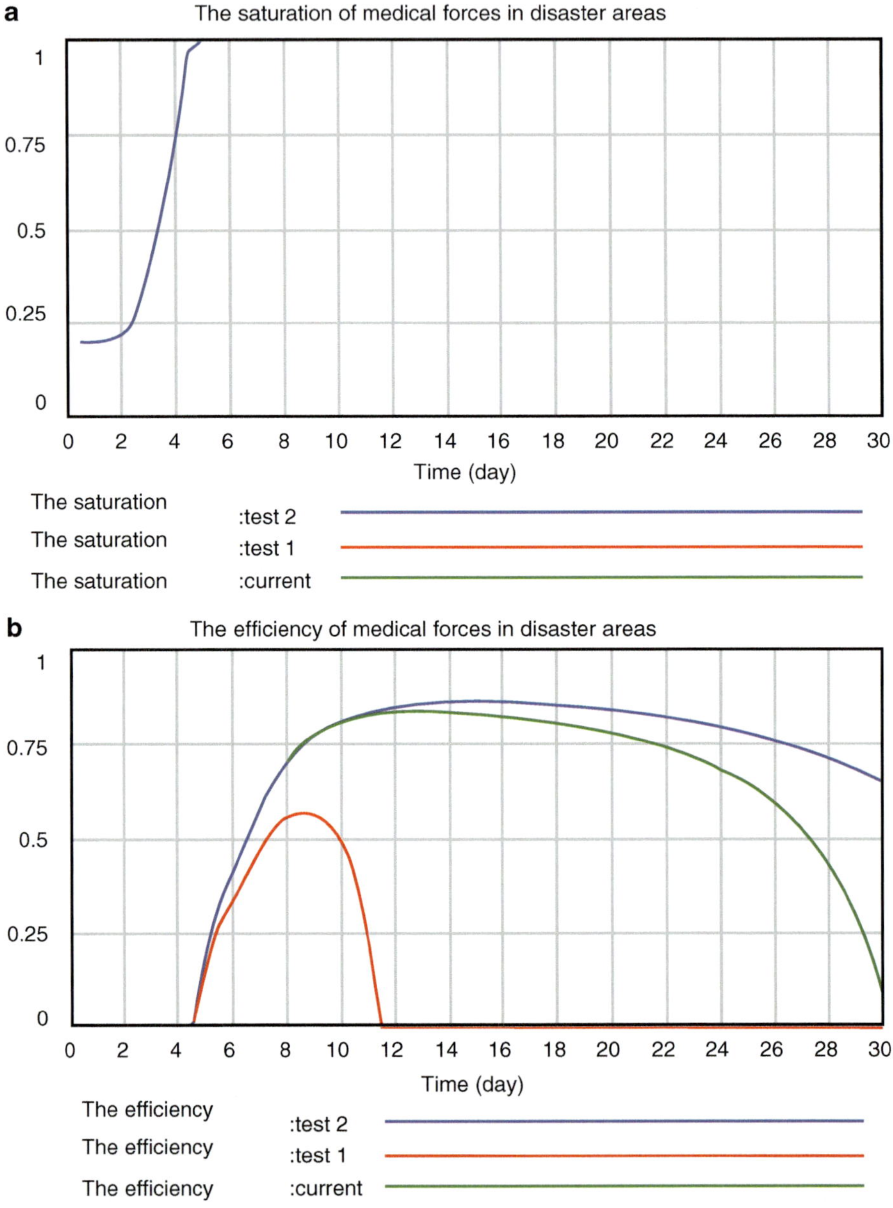

Fig. 4.11 Influence of different adjustment times of disaster medical forces in disaster areas on the system efficiency. (**a**) Variation of Medical forces saturation in disaster areas. (**b**) Variation of the efficiency of Medical forces in disaster areas

Adjusting the Initial Value of the Organization and Command Subsystem

To observe the influence of the initial value of the organization and command subsystem on treatment efficiency, three groups of intervention experiments were designed to conduct the model simulation.

Current: Adjusting the initial value of the sensitivity to the identification of treatment needs, the effectivity of medical evacuation plan, medical evacuation decision, and organization and command to 0.6

Test 1: Adjusting the initial value of the sensitivity to the identification of treatment needs, the effectivity of medical evacuation plan, medical evacuation decision, and organization and command to 0.1

Test 2: Adjusting the initial value of the sensitivity to the identification of treatment needs, the effectivity of medical evacuation plan, medical evacuation decision, and organization and command to 1

As shown in Fig. 4.12a, the initial value of need judge, medical evacuation plan, medical evacuation decision, and organization and command was adjusted in Test 2–1, which meant that the earthquake relief emergency preparation work was complete, organizing and command ability could exert itself completely, evacuation of the sick and wounded went smoothly, and the evacuation task could be completed in 3 days. Adjusting the initial value of need judge, medical evacuation plan, medical evacuation decision, and organization and command to 0.1 in Test 1 meant that earthquake relief emergency preparation work was not completed, organizing and command ability could not exert itself completely, and evacuation of the sick and wounded went slowly.

Figure 4.12b shows how the saturation of medical forces in the disaster areas changed, that is Test 2>Current>Test 1. This suggests that with better preparation, including adjusting the need judge, medical evacuation plan, medical evacuation decision, and organization and command, the drawing, deployment, and transportation could be completed much faster, which would allow the medical forces to arrive in disaster areas earlier to meet the treatment needs of the sick and wounded.

Figure 4.12c shows medical forces' low efficiency loss, Test 2>Current>Test 1. In other words, the improvement of adjusting the need judge, medical evacuation plan, medical evacuation decision, and organization and command could lead to the improvement of the macroscopical deployment, rapid decision adjustment, transportation, and retreat of the medical forces.

Earthquake relief and medical evacuation are emergency medical rescue tasks, which are conducted on certain intellectual and material foundations. The more sufficient the preparation in pacific times, the more sufficient medical forces, resource allocation, and the treatment and evacuation of the sick and wounded will be in times of crisis. Therefore, the improvement of the overall ability of the command system is key to improving the flexibility of the medical evacuation system. It will also make for better treatment and evacuation effectiveness and reduce resource waste.

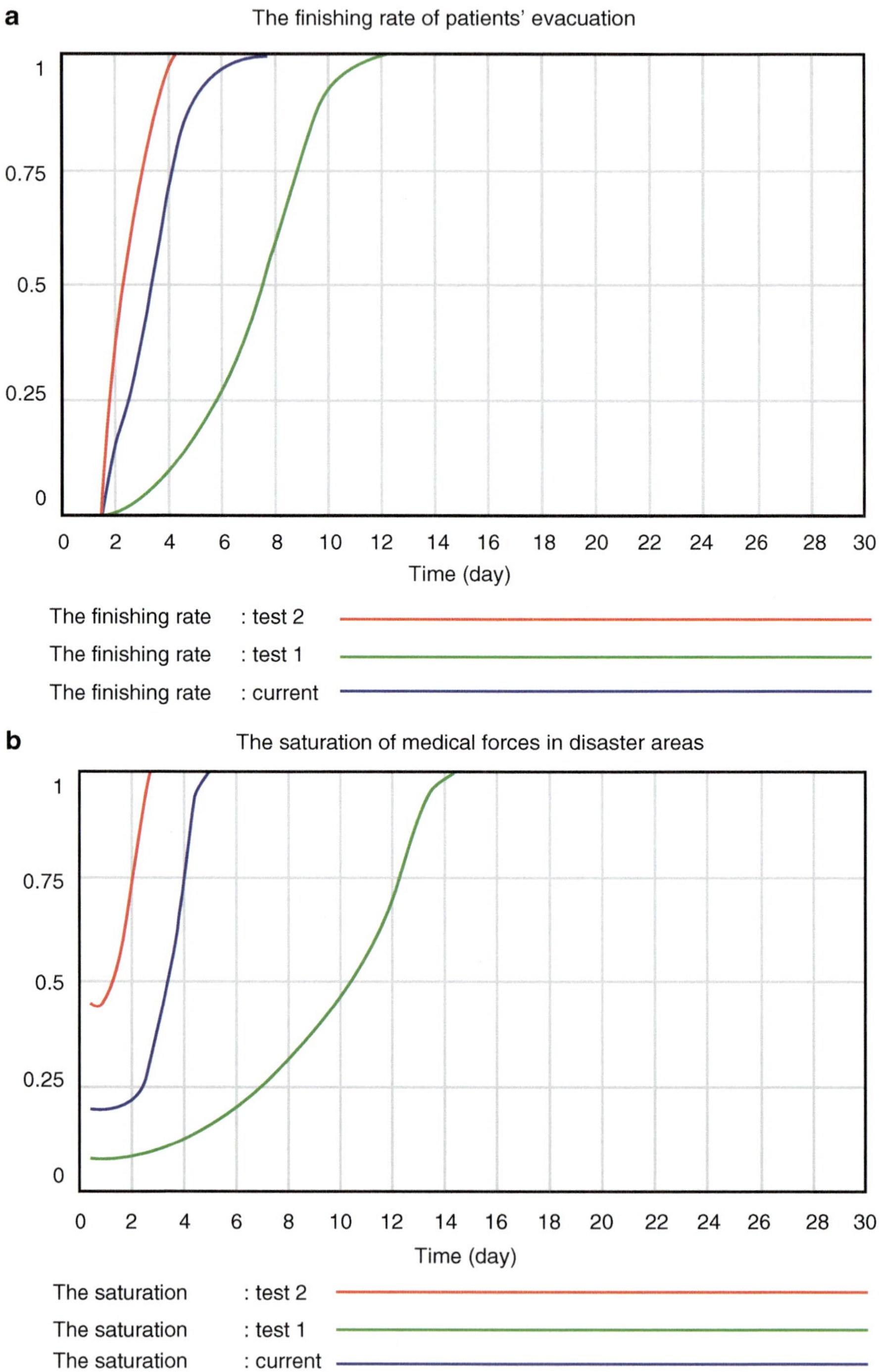

Fig. 4.12 Influence of adjusting the initial value of the organization and command sub-system on the system efficiency. (**a**) Variation of finishing rate of patients' evacuation. (**b**) (*Left*) variation of Medical forces saturation in disaster areas. (**c**) (*Right*) variation of the efficiency of Medical forces in disaster areas

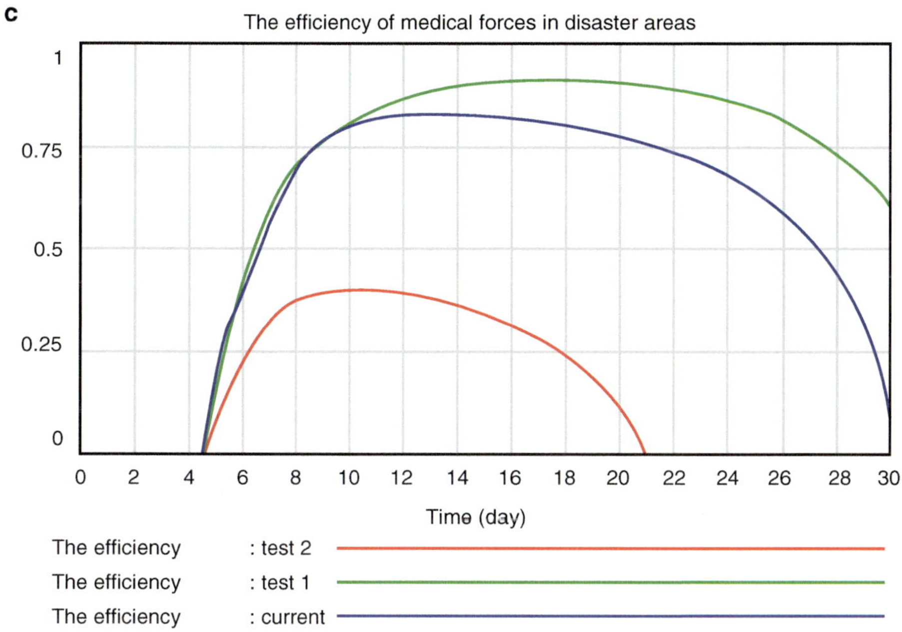

Fig. 4.12 (continued)

4.5 Summary

Evacuation velocity and resource utilization are often the key factors in earthquake relief and medical evacuation. Velocity and efficiency are significant characteristics of medical evacuation for earthquake relief. Evacuation velocity of the sick and wounded greatly affects medical evacuation growth; hence, rapid evacuation has become the main form of disaster medical rescue. In order to make the medical evacuation for earthquake relief faster and better, it would be necessary to improve evacuation velocity and medical resource utilization.

4.5.1 A Highly Sensitive Disaster Relief Emergency Command System Is a Precondition for Completing Disaster Relief Medical Evacuation

The key to enhancing medical evacuation efficiency for earthquake relief is to increase the efficiency of the emergency medical rescue organization and command. Sudden natural disasters like earthquakes require health departments to be ready in advance. Like the old saying "Maintain an army for a 1000 days to use it for an hour" urges, different rescue plans should be prepared in advance that consider the urgency, various demands, and complex environment of disaster medical relief tasks. Readiness of organization and command, information acquisition, medical personnel transfer, and a medical evacuation plan ought to be prepared according to the complexity. Many elements are important: strengthening emergency training, preparing in advance of an earthquake to lay a solid foundation of disaster emergency disposal, getting ready for an emergency dispatch and response, and ensuring that keen reaction and scientific deployment can be made under any condition.

The complexity of emergency disaster relief means that timely medical evacuation is strongly required. The quality and quantity of medical evacuations tend to change in a short period of time along with changes to external conditions. Successful evacuation preparation and implementation require more than evacuation plans and procedures.

Therefore, emergency medical rescue coordination agencies should improve their ability to deal with all kinds of problems in medical evacuation preparation and implementation. Comprehensive and focused preparation for earthquake disaster emergency medical relief should be organized and planned according to the needs of earthquake-prone areas and the reality of local health delivery systems in order to improve the commanding efficiency of medical evacuation.

A scientific and reasonable disaster relief emergency medical rescue mechanism with authority and effectiveness should be established. At the same time, a unified commanding organization joining military, police, and civilians is also needed. An improved linkage mechanism is required to enhance tight cooperation, the interaction of supply and demand, and the share of resources.

The following suggestions are important: improve the level of information, automate command means, perfect the medical evacuation plan, and optimize the evacuation plan. If there was more sufficient preparation, emergency medical relief after an earthquake could be initiated in a more confident, dynamic, and prompt manner (Shuai et al. 2004; Zong-chao 2008).

4.5.2 *Early Evacuation of the Sick and Wounded Would Help Shorten the Time That Patients Spend Moving from Injury to Specialized Treatment and Improve the Treatment Effect*

Earthquakes with a certain magnitude often cause the breakdown of medical service institutions that are located in epicenter areas. Rescue need, including specialist treatment, surgery, rehabilitation, and psychological support, would not be satisfied under such conditions.

Therefore, evacuating the sick and wounded to receive specialist treatment in rear hospitals has become one major mode of disaster emergency rescue. Early evacuation, specialist treatment, and rehabilitation are new trends in emergency medical rescues related to massive casualty incidents.

The earthquake commanding headquarters initiated trans-provincial evacuation of the sick and wounded. In all, 10,015 sick and wounded people were evacuated 6 days after the Wenchuan earthquake. Evacuation of the severely wounded in the Yushu earthquake was initiated on the first day of earthquake and was finished in 3 days. None of the severely wounded died in transit, and the overall death rate among the evacuated people was 0.10 %, which set a new record for safely evacuating the sick and wounded on the plateau.

4.5.3 The Proper Evacuation Ratio of the Sick and Wounded Has An Important Impact on Improving Medical Evacuation System Resource Utilization and Effectively Executing Classification Treatment

There are two emergency medical rescue organizing methods: (1) delivering large numbers of elite mobile medical forces to the front line for field first aid and (2) evacuating the sick and wounded in a timely fashion and safely to rear hospitals for treatments.

A proper evacuation ratio, which can be judged by the damage range, available medical forces in the disaster area, carrying capacity of evacuation carriers, and treatment needs, is key for improving the resource allocation efficiency of the medical evacuation system and effectively executing classification treatment.

Neglect of limited medical resources in disaster areas will cause a low evacuation ratio of the sick and wounded. This can lead to a situation in which the need for on-site treatments surpasses the medical service supply, which will keep the valid treatment rate relatively low. Furthermore, neglecting the carrying capacity of evacuation carriers will bring a high evacuation ratio of the sick and wounded, and a long waiting time for evacuation will delay specialist treatment.

In addition, an evacuation standard formulated from scientific and professional triage is of vital importance when there are limited medical resources after an earthquake. An ambiguous evacuation standard led to a situation in which more than 30 % of the wounded who were evacuated by helicopter from a particular disaster area were people who were wounded with minor injuries. Inappropriate triage and an indeterminate evacuation standard led simultaneously to waste and insufficient medical evacuation. Refining the standard of evacuation and adjusting the evacuation ratio according to the distribution of medical evacuation resources can rationalize the evacuation of the sick and wounded and help medical resources to be effectively utilized.

4.5.4 *Rational Allocation of Medical Forces in Disaster Areas and Rear Hospital Resources Is Key to Improving the System Efficiency of Earthquake Relief MES*

The low efficiency of medical forces in disaster areas that occurs 72 h after an earthquake could be avoided with timely adjustment. In the two on-site investigations we conducted, medical rescue commanders and team members agreed that the 24 h after an earthquake is a key period for medical rescue. Eight hours after an earthquake is a critical period of saving people. Specialists play a key role during the first 72 h and may be withdrawn after that time. Medical forces that stay should make their rounds as early as possible. Specialists could take turns supplementing the medical forces.

Medical forces began to retreat on the 9th day after the Yushu earthquake. All the supporting forces from other provinces, except military field shelter hospitals, retreated on the 17th day after the earthquake. On the 30th day, regional supporting forces retreated as well. Shelter hospitals provided medical services during the post-earthquake recovery and reconstruction, which was beyond the scope of the medical evacuation system. The deployment of medical forces for Yushu earthquake relief, compared with the retreat of medical forces 70 days after the Wenchuan earthquake, was more scientific and accorded with the occurrence characteristics of the sick and wounded.

The continuous medical needs of those being evacuated must be taken into consideration in choosing rear hospitals. The number of the sick and wounded peaked in 1 week and stayed at a high level for 2 weeks in most cases according to our research and literature review. The average length of in-hospital time was longer than usual. This was probably related to nonmedical causes such as post-earthquake arrangements. Commanding institutions should thoroughly assess the occupancy load when selecting rear hospitals. Rear hospitals should enhance their emergency management, properly arrange treatment for the sick and wounded, and estimate the need for rehabilitation and mental intervention.

To summarize, we can conclude from the model construction, simulation, and policy intervention experiment of the MES system dynamics model of earthquake relief that four aspects would help improve the velocity of evacuation and resource utilization and finally improve the overall effect of medical evacuation. They are the following: A. establishing a prepared and sensitive commanding system, B. early evacuation, C. a proper evacuation ratio, and D. coordinating to have enough mass rapid evacuation carriers.

References

Akbari ME, Farshad AA, Asadi-Lari M. The devastation of Bam: an overview of health issues 1 month after the earthquake. Public Health. 2004;118(6):403–8.

Chen J, Zhao W, Xian M, Lu J, Liang Z. Trans-Province Transfer of 10,373 Patients Injured in Wenchuan Earthquake. J Evidence-Based Med. 2009;2(4):270–6.

Kang P, Zhang L, Liang W, Zhu Z, Liu Y, Xu L, Yang H. Medical evacuation management and clinical characteristics of 3,255 inpatients after the 2010 Yushu earthquake in China. J Trauma Acute Care Surg. 2012;72(6):1626–33.

Liu X, Liu Y, Zhang L, Liang W, Zhu Z, Shen Y, Kang P, Liu Z. Mass aeromedical evacuation of patients in an emergency: experience following the 2010 yushu earthquake. J Emerg Med. 2013;45(6):865–71.

Nie H, Tang S-Y, Lau WB, Zhang J-C, Jiang Y-W, Lopez BL, Ma XL, Cao Y, Christopher TA. Triage during the week of the Sichuan earthquake: a review of utilized patient triage, care, and disposition procedures. Injury. 2011;42(5):515–20.

Shuai XH, Yang GL, Jiang LX. Earthquake disaster prevention and mitigation and emergency status in Japan. Earthquake (in Chinese). 2004;3:101–6.

Urbina E, Wolshon B. National review of hurricane evacuation plans and policies: a comparison and contrast of state practices. Transport Res Part A: Policy Pract. 2003;37(3):257–75.

Xiang B, Cheng W, Liu J, Huang L, Li Y, Liu L. Triage of pediatric injuries after the 2008 Wen-Chuan earthquake in China. J Pediatr Surg. 2009;44(12):2273–7.

Xu L, Lu-lu Z, Yuan L, Yi Z. Analysis and reflections on medical evacuation in Wenchuan Earthquake Relief. 2009;16(3):249–51.

Zhang L, Liu Y, Xu L, Zhang Y. Rescue efforts management and characteristics of casualties of the Wenchuan earthquake in China. Emerg Med J. 2011;28(7):618–22.

Zhang L, Xu L, Li Y, Liu Y, Liu Z, Lin J, Shen J, Tang X, Zhang Y, Liang W. Emergency medical rescue efforts after a major earthquake: lessons from the 2008 Wenchuan earthquake. Lancet. 2012;379(9818):853–61.

Zong chao P. An analysis on the governmental emergency responses to the Wenchuan massive earthquake in China. J China Execut Leader Acad Pudong. 2008;4:016.

Chapter 5
Modeling the Medical Rescue Forces Allocation in Earthquakes

Yuan Liu, Wenya Yu, Xu Liu, and Lulu Zhang

Abstract Medical rescue forces are the basis of earthquake rescue efforts. The allocation of medical rescue forces played vital role in the rescue efforts. This chapter mainly introduced the background, objective, significance, and technical route of medical rescue force allocation in earthquakes. The author described the process of the construction of medical rescue forces allocation model in earthquake. Based on the model construction, the systemic simulation and intervention were carried out so as to provide some suggestions on the allocation of medical rescue efforts.

5.1 Introduction to Medical Rescue Force Allocation in Earthquakes

5.1.1 Background

Earthquake medical rescue involves the complexity of subjects and elements, rigorous requirements of scientific decisions, and substantial difficulties with casualties forecasting, demands calculating, medical forces deployment, etc. Devastating earthquakes occur suddenly, and there is uncertainty with regard to the occurred time, area, intensity, and scope of the earthquake. These factors, coupled with the destruction of traffic, environment, and communications in earthquake-stricken areas, may lead the country or region into chaos. Thus, earthquake medical rescue teams must respond to extreme emergencies. It is impossible to plan and prepare in advance, and actions must often be taken immediately in the event of an emergency. Further, earthquakes require fast and efficient completion of the rescue mission. Earthquake medical rescue involves various tasks, including medical treatment,

Y. Liu, PhD • W. Yu • X. Liu, PhD
Department of Military Health Service, College of Military Health Service, Second Military Medical University, Yangpu, Shanghai, China

L. Zhang, PhD (✉)
Department of Military Health Service, College of Military Health Service, Second Military Medical University, Shanghai, China
e-mail: zllrmit@aliyun.com

© Springer Science+Business Media Dordrecht 2016

L. Zhang (ed.), *Modeling the Injury Flow and Treatment after Major Earthquakes*, DOI 10.1007/978-94-017-7527-4_5

epidemic prevention, and psychological rescue, in the face of a large number of victims, rescue workers, policy-makers, and so forth, with the need to coordinate logistics, communications, transportation, and other types of organizations. Moreover, the participating elements are diverse, the processes are complex, and the forms are various. Rapid deployment of rescue forces can greatly reduce casualties caused by earthquakes, and it is reported that in natural disasters, 20–30 % of the wounded and deceased can survive if they can have access to rapid treatment. Further, most of the victims may just be in need of the most basic medical care and treatment.

The medical and health demands after earthquakes show a clear staged process, and they can be divided into three stages: 24 h after the earthquake, 24 h to 2 weeks, and more than 2 weeks. The key points are significantly different across stages. The first stage emphasizes first aid, the second stage emphasizes epidemic prevention in disaster areas and evacuation transportation of the wounded for treatment, and the third stage mainly focuses on nosocomial infection control and rehabilitation therapy of casualties. Therefore, reasonable deployment of rescue forces, adjustment of rescue forces in time, and implementation of rescue mission conversion are directly related to the efficiency and even the success of the emergency medical rescue.

Earthquake emergency medical rescue forces are the structural foundation of the capabilities of earthquake emergency medical rescue, and scientific and rational deployment of rescue forces, timely adjustment of the deployment of rescue forces, and implementation of rescue mission conversion are directly related to the efficiency and success of emergency medical rescue. Further, most victims may need only the most basic medical care and treatment. Experiences from Wenchuan earthquake suggested that emergency medical rescue forces are not better with more numbers—disordered and blinded forces not only consume limited resources but also greatly increase the difficulty in organizing on-site treatment (Chen et al. 2012; Jiang et al. 2012). The key is to adjust the emergency medical rescue forces in time, and the transfer and deployment of emergency medical rescue forces should fit to the changing demands of the earthquake emergency medical rescue, thereby realizing the dynamic and optimal deployment of emergency medical rescue forces.

5.1.1.1 Current Situation of the Deployment of Earthquake Medical Rescue Abroad

The primary task of the earthquake emergency rescue is rescuing the wounded and patients! Take Wenchuan earthquake as an example: after the earthquake, the leader of the party and state always adheres to the principle of rescuing people first, not only to detect signs of survivors but also to fully treat those who had been injured. According to historical statistics, in the 1976 Tangshan earthquake, more than 8000 military health personnel were involved in the earthquake medical rescue, including 283 medical teams, 6 epidemic prevention teams, 5 field clinics, and 3 field hospitals. In the 2008 Wenchuan earthquake, there were more than 50,000 frontline medical staff directly participating in medical rescue in disaster areas, including 5969 medical personnel from various provinces of the country, 7061 military health personnel, 244 foreign and regional rescue personnel, and 41,240 people of medical institutions at all levels in Sichuan Province. Ultimately, more than 200 million wounded people were rescued and treated. Earthquake emergency medical rescue includes not only the rescue and treatment of the sick and wounded but also epidemic prevention, psychological rescue, and the protection of medicines and materials in disaster areas. In the Wenchuan earthquake medical rescue, a cumulative total of 1.14 billion square meters environment were sterilized, 974,300 houses and tents were provided, and 149,100 people received psychological counseling. In the 2010 Yushu earthquake, the country and the army sent more than 5000 medical staff, and it can be seen from the rescue and treatment of the wounded; the tasks of earthquake emergency medical rescue are substantial and play an irreplaceable role in earthquake rescue (Chen et al. 2012; Jiang et al. 2012; Liu et al. 2012; Zhang et al. 2012; Zhang et al. 2011).

In the 1976 Tangshan earthquake rescue, due to the limited medical technologies and means of communication means, among other factors, some of the wounded were disabled or died on account of a lack of timely and effective treatment. In the Wenchuan earthquake medical rescue, among medical staff sent by the army were individuals holding a masters or doctoral degree, who accounted for more than 70 % of the staff in a group of experts led by several academicians, all of whom showed a high level of knowledge of current technologies for earthquake emergency medical rescue. Accordingly, failed rescue due to defects in medical technologies rarely occurred. Today, medical technologies have been highly developed, and it seems that the needs of emergency medical rescue can be satisfied as long as there is a sufficient amount of rescue forces. However, the principles of scientific management suggest that only superior resources and scientific and effective decision-making can play a significant role. Experiences with the Wenchuan earthquake also suggest that emergency medical rescue forces are not better with numbers, as disordered and blinded forces not only consume limited resources but also greatly increase the organization difficulty of on-site treatment. For example, within 24 h of the Wenchuan earthquake, a large amount of medical rescue forces were concentrated on the epicenter, but because of the restrictions of the geographical environment, the entrance of rescue forces was blocked, causing a lot of retention. This resulted in an inability to deploy in time as well as a wasted opportunity to enter the area and provide access to medical rescue and treatment, thereby reducing the overall efficiency of the emergency medical rescue (Jiang et al. 2012; Zhang et al. 2008, 2011). The key is that they did not adjust the decisions regarding emergency medical rescue in a timely matter, resulting in disordered and blinded support. This was also a manifestation of the deficiency of the emergency medical rescue organization decision-making, and thus it cannot be ignored that the improper decision-making of emergency medical rescue organization led to inefficient rescue. The rational use of earthquake medical rescue forces is the core of decision-making regarding earthquake emergency medical rescue, and thus, the theoretical study of earthquake emergency medical rescue is a crucial issue that must be addressed.

In the Bam earthquake, medical rescue forces of Iran were mainly based on military forces. The army began to rescue the wounded within 1 h after the disaster and established Iran's first local field hospital in disaster areas (Abolghasemi et al. 2005).

On the day of the earthquake, the army transported 937 medical and healthcare staff and assistants to the disaster area, established 23 field emergency clinics and 13 field rescue centers, and ran eight rescue centers in rear hospitals across the country. To ensure an adequate supply of medical materials and necessities, the Iranian military sent 185 rescue teams with a total number of 1286 people, and the rescue personnel included healthcare staff and medical staff. Medical staff included general practitioners, medical specialists, public health personnel, and primary healthcare personnel, and these individuals were pre-programmed in the military medical institutions. Meanwhile, the military of Iran established two field hospitals, 23 field emergency clinics, and 13 rescue centers and provided the necessary medical materials and equipment (Abolghasemi et al. 2005). The military of Iran established rehabilitation centers based on eight rear hospitals, and each of them was equipped with specialized surgeons.

A few hours after the Bam earthquake, the US government immediately sent a Boston-based international surgical response team to the disaster areas. The surgical response team included 58 medical staff, including specialists in trauma surgery, obstetrics and gynecology, anesthesiology, primary care, pediatrics, and emergency medicine, as well as medical support staff and nurses, all of whom were from the emergency departments, operating rooms, and intensive care units and, finally, some pharmacy and logistic staff. All staff with full installation mobilized to the disaster areas within 12 h, and there were expanded field hospitals near the four international field hospitals of Ukraine, France, Spain, and Norway.

After the Yogyakarta earthquake in Indonesia, the US military deployed medical and logistic staff in the worst affected district, Bantul, within 72 h. The rescue team included the US military third Okinawa-based maritime expeditionary brigade in Japan, Mercy hospital ship, and some naval personnel, totaling 286 individuals (Amundson et al. 2008). The Mercy hospital ship provided professionals of internal medicine, pediatrics, and general and preventive medicine, thereby strengthening the medical treatment of the third maritime expeditionary brigade. A traumatic shock treatment platoon from the ship simultaneously joined the medical rescue team, totaling 37 medical staff. The third maritime expeditionary brigade provided basic laboratory equipment (including blood count, blood gas analysis, and urine analysis instruments) as well as a portable X-ray machine.

In the Haiti earthquake, the Israeli government promptly sent military medical forces with 230 people to the disaster area and established a fully functional field hospital 89 h after the earthquake in disaster areas (Merin et al. 2010; Liu et al. 2014). The field hospital had 60 beds, four intensive care units, and an operating room. In addition to large amounts of commonly used drugs, diagnostic imaging equipment, clinical laboratory equipment, and sterilization equipment, the hospital was allocated with power generation equipment and life support facilities, all deployed from Israel by air, thus ensuring a strong self-protection capacity (Bilham 2010).

Studies about the earthquake emergency medical rescue forces both domestically and abroad mainly center on the medical and health demands after disasters and conduct related research regarding rescue forces. It can be seen from the practice of international medical teams participating in earthquake emergency medical rescues of other countries that foreign emergency medical rescue forces showed some advantages in terms of high mobility, strong self-protection, and fast response time. The stages of foreign earthquake emergency medical rescues are consistent with our research group's findings, and differences are mainly on the start and end times of each stage. That is, the duration of each stage is different. Compared with some related foreign studies, it is essential to determine whether the characteristics of the Wenchuan earthquake emergency medical rescue forces have universal significance and whether we can establish basic guidelines for transfer and deployment of emergency medical rescue forces.

5.1.2 Objective and Significance

The deployment of earthquake medical rescue forces occurs in accordance with complex adaptive systems (CAS) theory, using methods like systems analysis, literature meta-induction, and multi-body modeling through the retrospective analysis of earthquake emergency medical rescue both domestically and abroad. Systematic analyses were conducted on the deployment of earthquake medical rescue forces to establish a multi-agent system model of the deployment of earthquake medical rescue forces. We also explored the relationships among the bodies of forces, decision-making, and the object in earthquake medical rescue, and through empirical analyses of the efficiency and results of the deployment of medical rescue forces in Wenchuan and Yushu earthquakes, we determined the underlying rules of the deployment of earthquake medical rescue forces.

Based on the empirical analysis of the human resource allocation for the Yushu earthquake medical rescue, we determined the total amount and distribution characteristics of human resource allocation in earthquake medical rescues, as well as the change disciplines of the internal structure, thus providing a scientific basis for the scientific, rational, and efficient deployment of earthquake medical rescue forces.

5.1.3 Technical Route and Design

The microscopic behaviors of the deployment of earthquake medical rescue forces allowed for the emergence of the system that is the so-called small property generates big behavior, where changes in the properties and states of microscopic strength cause macroscopic changes in the system's performance. Under the theoretical framework of the early logistic decision support studies of the research group, and based on the ideology of multi-agent modeling of complex adaptive systems, this study is a basic application study aiming to discover the evolution process and characteristics of the deployment system for earthquake medical rescue forces by analyzing the behavior disciplines of each body of the earthquake medical rescue forces. Ultimately, we will provide earthquake medical rescue forces with guidelines for scientific, rapid, and efficient deployment.

This section focuses on complex problems of the deployment of earthquake medical rescue forces. Based on the defined studies on the deployment of medical rescue forces and systematic analyses of the deployment of medical rescue forces from a multi-agent perspective, this study formed a research idea of the deployment of medical rescue forces based on multi-agent systems. Moreover, through the main concept models and multi-agent interaction models of the deployment of earthquake medical rescue forces, this section conducted empirical analyses on the deployment of the Wenchuan and Yushu earthquake medical rescue forces and determined the laws, characteristics, and system evolution process involved.

5.2 Data Resource Used in Medical Rescue Forces Allocation in Earthquakes

The relevant data on the deployment of earthquake medical rescue forces are all from the practices of Wenchuan and Yushu earthquake medical rescues. The key points include data regarding medical rescue teams at different levels, organizational headquarters, and the treatment of the sick and wounded. Specific contents include the number of sick and wounded individuals being treated. The medical staff survey in Yushu County mainly addresses medical rescue behaviors within 72 h, situations of participating in supporting forces, views on the utilization and deployment of supporting forces, and so on. In the expert consultation and demonstration meetings, we counseled the key factors influencing the deployment of earthquake medical rescue forces and behavior rules of the main bodies (Xiao-Ming 2012; Yuan et al. 2011).

5.2.1 Utilization of the Current Data Resource

This study mainly used the following data: (1) basic information from previous earthquakes, mainly information collected from the Internet; (2) over 20 relevant studies on foreign earthquake medical rescue retrieved from the databases PubMed, Elsevier, Tsinghua Tongfang CNKI, and Chongqing VIP; (3) over 100 copies of related documents, reports, and statistics on the Yushu earthquake emergency medical rescue from the National Ministry of Health; (4) collections of more than 80 copies of documents from the health department of the Department of Joint Logistics of Chengdu Military Region and the Second Military Medical University of Wenchuan earthquake rescue newsletters and more than 20 copies of relevant documents; and (5) collection of 20 copies of Yushu earthquake rescue newsletters of the health department of Joint Logistics Department of Lanzhou Military Region and more than 10 copies of relevant documents.

5.2.2 *Data Source from Field Survey*

The data sources mainly include on-site survey data of Wenchuan and Yushu earthquakes.

5.2.2.1 Time and Objects of Investigation

The research group conducted 10 days of on-site research in the Wenchuan earthquake disaster area since June 13, 2008. Based on a focus analysis of the earthquake medical rescue by Second Military Medical University, the research group conducted a sample survey of the military earthquake medical rescue action and investigated the situation of the wounded in the hardest-hit areas of Mianyang, Mianzhu and Dujiangyan, Pengzhou, Beichuan, An County, Mao County, and Yingxiu town. The objects of the investigation are mainly medical rescue agencies and medical rescue headquarters. The research group investigated the military medical rescue headquarters at all levels, including medical rescue squad command, frontline command of the major units, command in responsible areas, joint command in the region of wars, and the general logistics working group. We also investigated various types of military and civilian medical rescue agencies, including the strategic support medical rescue squad, medical rescue squad sent by different military regions, the logistic squad of organic military, and the medical rescue squad in Chengdu Military Region. The categories included medical teams, epidemic prevention teams, psychological rescue teams, seven field hospitals (two square cabin-style field hospitals), rear hospitals in disaster areas, and the medical institutions in local areas as well as those supported by other countries.

The research group conducted a 1-week on-site earthquake survey in Yushu, Xining, and Qinghai in December 2010 and subsequently conducted supplementary research in Sichuan, Shanxi, Gansu, and Tibet Autonomous Region. The objects of the investigation were mainly medical rescue agencies, health administrations, and medical rescue personnel. The survey investigated health administrative agencies, namely, the Qinghai Provincial Health Department Emergency Management Office, Bureau of Medical Affairs, and Yushu Prefecture Health Bureau. (During the investigation, the relevant personnel were being trained in Xining training.) We also investigated medical and health institutions supported by Yushu in Qinghai Province, including more than 10 units, such as the Qinghai Provincial People's Hospital, affiliated hospital of Qinghai University, Qinghai Red Cross Hospital, People's Armed Police Corps Hospital of Qinghai Province, and Qinghai Province Center for Disease Control and Prevention (Jiang et al. 2010; Kang et al. 2012; Liu et al. 2012).

5.2.2.2 Survey Methods

The survey mainly used interviews, small-scale meetings, and focus group interviews. The interview outlines were set in each interview. More than 50 frontline medical experts and medical rescue leaders from different levels were interviewed;

over 10 small-scale forums, which included rear hospitals, medical rescue squads, and medical rescue commanding officers of all levels, were held. This spanned three focus group interviews on the given topics. The interview results were recorded in the form of text and audio, and the data were organized after the research. Further, and the forum acted as a brainstorming session for medical rescue experts. During the interviews, the research group members and interviewed people were all allowed to submit problems arising from medical rescue actions, and during the interviews, these problems were discussed and analyzed, and solutions were proposed. Investigations mainly focused on medical staff participating in earthquake emergency medical rescue, including more than 300 medical staff in Qinghai Province and over 120 medical staff in Yushu. The supplementary investigation in Sichuan, Shanxi, Gansu, and Tibet Autonomous Region mainly took the form of telephone and network surveys, and the surveys were handed over to the health department by the research group members. The health departments of the four provinces were responsible for completing the questionnaires and tables, and the relevant data were sent back to the research group.

5.2.2.3 Survey Content

The survey content was set according to the objects of investigation. The survey of health administrative agencies included the command system, institutional levels, establishment time, coordination mechanisms, and the utilization of forces. The survey of medical treatment institutions included the number and the sources of the wounded being treated, medical evacuation system, situation of mobility, situation of deployment, and situation of mobility. The survey of medical staff in Qinghai Province included the general situation of the staff and the medical treatment situation. The survey of medical staff in Yushu County included the medical rescue behaviors within 72 h, situations of participating in supporting forces, views on the utilization and deployment of the supporting forces, and so on. In the expert consultation and demonstration meetings, we counseled the key factors influencing the deployment of earthquake medical rescue forces and behavior rules of the agents including casualties, medical forces, and decision-makers.

5.2.2.4 Quality Control

During interviews, the research group drafted detailed outlines through meticulous data collection, communicated and discussed problems in accordance with the outlines one by one, and extensively listened to the views and opinions of interviewees and conference members, which were all recorded and arranged by research group members. Before conducting questionnaire surveys, the research group members emphasized the significance of the survey in detail and explained the key subjects in turn, thus ensuring the quality of the questionnaires completed by subjects. In the survey of the local medical staff in Yushu County, the investigation was coordinated with the staff of the local health bureau, who interpreted each questionnaire question, thus avoiding problems that might be caused by language differences.

In addition, some research group members conducted an on-site investigation in Yushu disaster areas in April 2010 and collected some related documents of the Ministry of Health Joint Logistics Department in Lanzhou Military Region, thereby providing data support for subjects' interviews and surveys. In October 2010, the research group collected relevant literature on the Yushu earthquake emergency medical rescues from the National Ministry of Health, mainly involving daily information on the duties of National Ministry of Health during the Yushu earthquake emergency medical rescue, as well as documents of the mobility of the medical rescue forces and some related policies and documents.

5.2.3 *Collection of Documents*

The research group consulted more than ten types of related articles in professional journals from 1997 to 2011, such as *Medical Service Journal of Chinese People's Liberation Army*, *Hospital Management Journal of Chinese People's Liberation Army*, *Journal of System Simulation*, and *Medicine of Chinese People's Liberation Army*. Using both manual selection and Medline to select articles, we selected more than 80 articles that referred to earthquake rescue, earthquake emergency medical rescue, and multi-agent modeling.

5.3 Construction of Medical Rescue Forces Allocation Model in Earthquake

5.3.1 *Definitions of the Agents of Medical Rescue Forces Allocation in Earthquake*

5.3.1.1 Agent Classification of the System

In the system of medical rescue forces allocation during earthquakes, there are three agent categories: forces (earthquake medical rescue forces), decision-making (medical rescue command and decision-making institutions), and objects (rescued objects, mainly referring to the sick and wounded). Each agent can change its behaviors according to information provided by the system.

The force agents mainly include medical rescue forces and health and epidemic prevention forces; the decision-making agents mainly include medical rescue agencies of strategy, campaign, and tactics; and the rescued object agents are the sick and wounded individuals in disaster areas. Interactions between agents occur through the function of the environment, and the treatment for the sick and wounded of a certain force agent will affect the behaviors of the other forces. Among the three types of agents, further distinction between the intelligent and non-intelligent agents is necessary. Intelligent agents generally have a goal and can perceive the environment and make decisions based on partial information or respond to external stimulations. Non-intelligent individuals can only react passively. Further, there are partial agents whose intelligence lies somewhere between the two types. Therefore, the core of the decision-making agents is the policy-makers, who are the intelligent bodies, and the object agents are also intelligent bodies. The force agents change their behaviors according to the requirements of decision-making agents and can also make decisions autonomously, which are between the intelligent and non-intelligent bodies, and the environmental agents can be seen as non-intelligent bodies. Based on multi-agent system characteristics, for the force agents, the decision-making bodies may be their behavioral environment, which provides environmental infrastructure for the interactions among objects included in the various types of agents.

5.3.1.2 Property and Status of the System Agents

1. The properties of the force agents include the existence of classification, rank, quantity, morbidity time, deployment forms, deployment time, deployment location, treatment capacity, quality, and load. The deployment forms can be divided into separate modules, sub-detachments, module systems, and mixed groups. Categories include medical and epidemic prevention classes. Levels are divided into strategic, regional, and local, and loads are split into full, free, and medium.
2. The properties of the decision-making agents include level, decision-making content, and decision-making time. The levels include strategic, campaign, and tactics, and decision-making contents include the objects, times, and quantities of force mobility and deployment.
3. The properties of the object agents include status, location, quantity, and outcome. Statuses include being treated and not being treated by medical rescue forces. Outcomes include improvement, recovery, disability, and death.

5.3.2 Conceptual Model of the Agents of Medical Rescue Force Allocation During Earthquakes

5.3.2.1 Conceptual Model of the Force Agents of Medical Rescue Force Allocation During Earthquakes

Evolution of Agents

The conceptual model of the force agents was built according to the characteristics of medical rescue forces' mobility and allocation during an earthquake. Take the medical forces as an example: the decision-making agent will make decisions about

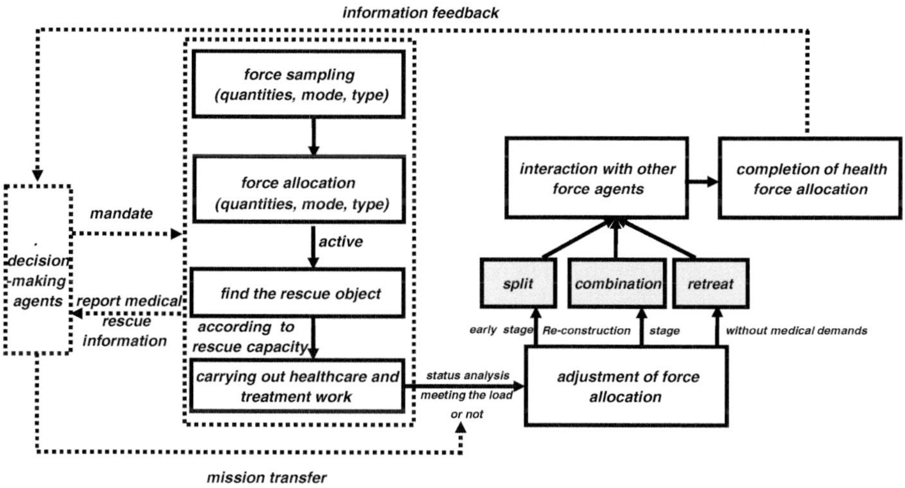

Fig. 5.1 Evolution process of the forces agents of medical rescue in earthquakes

medical rescue mobility after the analysis of the environment and demand of the earthquake. Medical rescue forces will be allocated to designated areas and take treatment actions for the sick and the wounded. After medical rescue force agents arrive at the designated mission areas, the main task is to treat the sick and the wounded, and the specific methods include receiving and evacuating the sick and wounded and actively accepting them at the frontline. During the process of treating the sick and the wounded, it is necessary to submit treatment information to decision-making agents on time. Meanwhile, it is also necessary to change the allocation patterns according to the actual treatment situation of the sick and the wounded and the stages of the entire emergency medical rescue operation (Fig. 5.1). If the wounded are not received in a certain time, forces must consider changing the allocation location or the allocation forms, and treat the sick and the wounded by splitting units or retreating according to commands. Medical rescue teams can allocate in accordance with splitting and/or combination, and in this process, along with interacting with the other force agents, teams can achieve the goals of the medical rescue forces allocation system in earthquakes through optimal allocation of personnel, equipment, and materials.

According to the conclusions of qualitative system analysis, this study distinguished the behaviors of medical rescue forces in earthquakes using different allocation positions and methods representing various medical rescue force behaviors. Based on the emergency decision plans of decision-making agents and combined with their own rescue and protection levels, medical rescue forces can realize optimal utilization of their own resources. Their behavioral characteristics are mainly represented as different medical rescue demands for mobility and allocation of different types of medical rescue forces, and the indexes include the time, quantity, method, and quality of mobility and allocation. Finally, the main influencing factors include their establishment, capability, geographic environment, and occurrence disciplines of the sick and the wounded in disaster areas.

Behavior Rules of Agents

After an earthquake, medical forces quickly concentrate in the disaster areas and are allocated given the circumstances of the wounded. Relevant studies abroad also suggest that the utilization of military medical rescue forces in earthquake should follow two basic elements. First, the rapid utilization of local military forces of disaster areas, and second, the rapid transportation of medical rescue forces needed outside of the disaster areas. Medical rescue force allocation must be rapid, and the mobility and allocation time is an important indicator. The quantity of medical force allocation is closely related to the assessment results of decision-making agents, and the quantity changes of decision-making agents are all based on the official information reports. Medical forces only interact with the adjacent forces, specifically engaging in cooperation and combination. When the quantity of the sick and the wounded received is more than the receiving capacity, it is necessary to evacuate to the nearest medical forces, and if it is beyond the capacity of the nearest medical treatment area, to continue searching. Medical teams are allocated with 50 staff, and they mainly conduct emergency treatment and early treatment, completing the treatment of 120–140 wounded people day and night. When the quantity properties of the object agents reach 80 % of the total treatment capacity of medical forces, the properties of the force agents should transformed. When the increasing index number of object agents is less than a certain threshold, the force agents show a free or medium load, and the medical force agents change the property of the allocation mode and begin to split into detachments for rounds of visits. Each detachment is allocated with five staffs, who make their rounds of visits once a day, with two groups being sent daily. Their own behaviors as force agents include treatment of the wounded, acceptance of the participation of local medical staff, and combination and mixing with other medical forces. When the rescue efforts enter into the reconstruction stage, medical and epidemic prevention forces may all retreat or form a new medical treatment system to complete the daily medical and health demands of the affected areas by modular combination.

5.3.2.2 Conceptual Model of Decision-Making Agents of Medical Rescue Force Allocation During Earthquakes

Evolution of Agents

After the earthquake, decision-making agents should analyze the situation rapidly, organize the mobility of medical rescue forces, and determine the mobility methods, quantities, and resources according to casualties reported by the earthquake areas as well as information obtained from other sources. In accordance with the progress of medical rescue actions, decision-making agents should supplement and adjust medical rescue forces at any time and determine the allocation position, methods, and retreatment times of medical rescue forces. After the initial information gathering and decision-making, decision-making agents will determine the

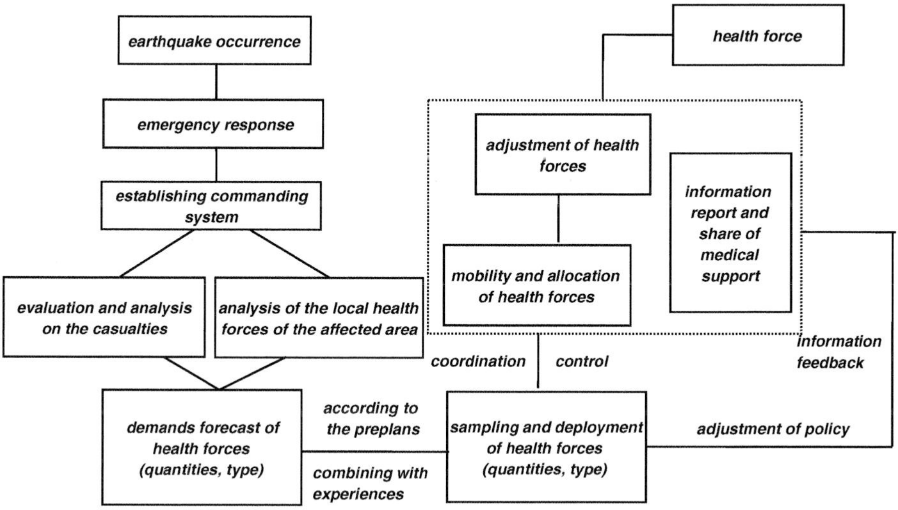

Fig. 5.2 Evolution process of decision-making agents in medical rescue forces allocation

allocation of medical forces and the health and epidemic prevention forces to a certain mission area. Through coordination and control, medical rescue forces assume a certain mobility method to reach mission areas to launch their allocation (Fig. 5.2). In addition, decision-making agents should collect and analyze the situations of casualties and treatment of the sick and the wounded in a timely manner and propose relevant policies and recommendations for medical rescue force allocation according to the phase characteristics of the medical rescue actions and changes in the overall environment.

Decisions regarding medical rescue forces allocation are typical emergency decisions whose organization foundation is the establishment of a health organizational headquarters at all levels. The medical rescue organization and command system must adhere to the principles of commanding in the frontlines and keep the system flat, thus improving the operating efficiency of the organization.

Behavior Rules of Agents

Based on the system theories and emergency decision-making process, the medical rescue force allocation decision system can be divided into four subsystems: decision-making goals, decision-making constraints, decision-making centers, and the implementation of decision-making. The four subsystems interact with each other, affected by the influences of environment, resources, and policies, as well as through information exchanges and established decision-making mechanisms, which promote the development of the decision-making process regarding medical rescue force allocation. By exploring the behavioral rules of decision-making agents, we can analyze the four subsystems of medical rescue force allocation decision system.

The medical rescue force allocation decision system includes casualties, rescue time, resource efficiency, and so forth, which are the bases of the formulation and implementation of the force allocation programs, and plays a decisive role in the formation of the medical rescue force allocation plan and is also an important evidence of the assessment of the effect of force allocation decisions. The determination or adjustment of medical rescue force allocation decision goals should be based on processes and implementation effects of the medical rescue actions and are closely related to the extent of the earthquake's damage and the development stages of overall rescue actions. For example, the goal of the emergency medical rescue phase is generally to maximize the treatment of lives, and the later decision goal also includes ensuring that the disaster areas are free from mass infectious diseases.

The constraint systems of medical rescue force allocation decisions include elements of supplies of drugs, medical rescue forces, information and management, and medical technologies. The primary task of earthquake rescue is to save people, and resource demands have a strong sense of urgency and dynamic timeliness, which need to be adjusted in accordance with the process of emergency medical rescue actions and dynamic multistage adjustment of the previous stage of the rescue effects. The internal and external environments of medical rescue actions change dramatically, often resulting in a scarcity of key local resources and information. For example, strong aftershocks and secondary disasters will lead to a lack of regional medical rescue forces or a shortage of medicines and equipment, as well as difficulties in information sharing among decision-making agents at all levels because of a partial breakdown in communications. Based on the complex adaptive characteristics of the medical rescue force allocation system, the evolution process of its emergency decision also has complex features and is simultaneously constrained by the emergency response mechanism and technical level.

The central system of the medical rescue force allocation decision system is the core of the decision system, which has decision-making authorization, issuing orders and decision support functions, and has a coordination and control role of the operation of the entire force allocation system. The central system includes the decision-making agents, assisting decision-making institutions, and plan libraries. The complexity of the medical rescue force allocation necessarily makes its emergency decision-making a process of expert group decision-making. Assisting decision-making institutions provides the entire decision-making system with supporting methods and decision-making suggestions, and based on studies on decision-making mechanisms and evaluation methods, they actualize the medical rescue force allocation plan system, provide decision recommendations about scientific force allocations, and deal with the ex post evaluation of the emergency decision effects.

The implementation system of medical rescue force allocation is a system that can bring about specific behaviors of established plans and projects and particularly the behaviors of force agents. The implementation of disposal is a process of playing the decision function under the coordination and control of the central decision system, as well as under the influences of the target and restraint systems. According to the progress of medical rescue actions, and the differences in the quantity and quality of medical rescue forces, agents involved in the specific medical rescue forces are different.

5.3.2.3 Conceptual Model of the Object Agents of Medical Rescue Force Allocation During Earthquakes

Evolution of Agents

The object agents are the individuals being rescued after the earthquake. After the earthquake, the injured individuals will call for help and self-help, and those who are discovered by the force agents will receive medical treatment. Individuals being treated have four outcomes: improvement, recovery, disability, and death. Objects recovered may also join with the force agents and participate in medical rescue actions as volunteers. In addition, the situation of local medical rescue forces after the earthquake deserves further attention, as these individuals will often become the main source of medical rescue forces. Behaviors of rescued objects affect the properties and states of the medical rescue forces. For instance, the rescued object agents with infectious diseases will emphasize the provision of health epidemic prevention. The rescued objects utilize various medical services provided by force agents to realize self-diagnosis of their own injuries, treatment and prevention, and improve their health conditions. Their behavior characteristics are mainly represented in the changes of states of the sick and wounded after being treated by different medical rescue forces. After being treated by the force agents, the object agents decrease appreciably from an increase state and ultimately maintain a steady state. The status evolution of the object agents is mainly influenced by the discovery time, the level of the force agents, the discovery location, and the transportation situation (Fig. 5.3).

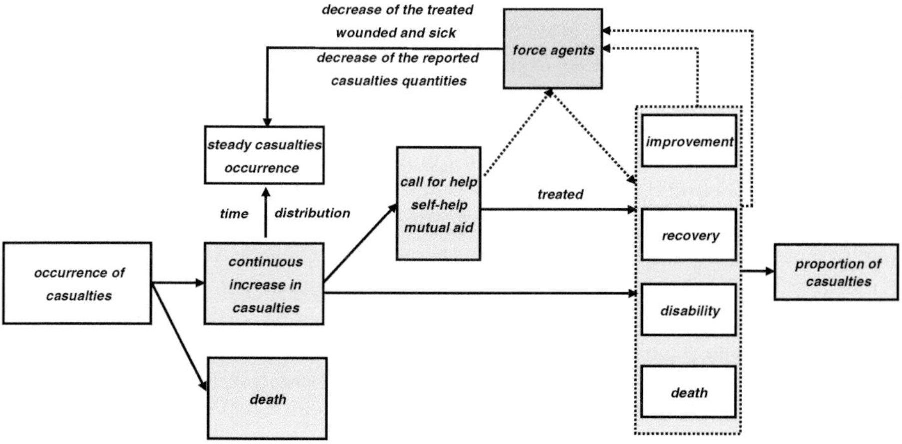

Fig. 5.3 Evolution process of object agents in medical rescue forces allocation

Behavior Rules of Agents

The generating law disciplines of casualties in earthquakes are always difficult to determine for earthquake rescue studies, as most of the studies propose factors that influence casualties, including the magnitude, building structure, time of occurrence, focal depth, pre-earthquake prediction, and natural environment in earthquake areas. Thus far, however, there exists no reasonable prediction model. It can be found from the study that the occurrence time of casualties in earthquakes, spatial distributions, and analyses of proportions of casualties have a reference value for the demand prediction and rescue actions of the medical rescue in earthquakes. Some scholars have studied the reported times of the number of deaths in earthquakes and found that these reported times of the number of deaths are associated with the total number of deaths. Rescue personnel rescue the trapped in the rubble, need to clean and search every house, and rescuing survivors and discovering victims are carried out simultaneously. The number of deaths and injuries both have a good correlation with the presented curves of their reported times. The more deaths, the longer the time needed for rescue and the later the reported time will be. The shorter the reported time of the number of deaths becomes close to the total number of deaths, the more clearly the outside world will understand the earthquake; the earlier into the disaster areas will come the rescue personnel and rescue materials, the more quickly the disordered status of the disaster areas can be restored and the stronger the rescue capabilities will be. The time allowed for digging out buried people after earthquakes is limited, as survival time underneath the rubble is limited, and the longer the digging time, the slimmer the survival hopes become. If the reported time is late, the outside world will not understand the actual facts of the situation, and it becomes difficult for the earthquake rescue headquarters to mobilize enough rescue personnel and provide abundant materials. Consequently, disaster areas will lack outside aid, and the disordered state will be extended.

Implementation of emergency treatment for the sick and wounded within the 72-h "golden rescue period" after the earthquake can effectively reduce mortality and morbidity. It turns out that digging the wounded from the rubble within 24 h with timely treatment can effectively reduce the number of deaths. According to the statistics of a Tangshan earthquake rescue army, digging within half an hour can save 90.4 % of buried victims, whereas digging in the first day can save 81.0 %, and digging in the second day can save 33.0 %. Digging in the fourth day, however, can only save 19.0 %. Practices both domestically and abroad all show that the survival rate of early rescue is high, and the survival rate of late rescue declines sharply, and through several retrospective analyses of earthquakes, it can be found that the survival rate of the wounded is a function of the time after earthquakes. Therefore, rapid, timely, and accurate utilization of forces is the key to reducing casualties, which fully reflects the close relationship between characteristics of the decision-making agents and the agents.

5.3.3 *Multi-Agent Model Framework of Medical Rescue Force Allocation During Earthquakes*

According to the rules, agents generate behaviors and interact with each other. The behavior designation of interactions between agents should not be too complex, as long as it can reflect the basic principles of the real system, and can determine the evolution characteristics of the system through interactions.

5.3.3.1 Multi-Agent Interaction Framework of Medical Rescue Force Allocation During Earthquakes

It can be found from the analysis of the evolution and behavior rules of various agents of medical rescue in earthquakes that behaviors of force agents include implementation of medical treatment, implementation of health and epidemic prevention, adjustment of force allocation methods, change of force allocation location, and transfer of medical rescue information. Behaviors of decision-making agents include force mobility, order of force allocation instructions, establishment of rescue mechanisms, policy-making, and information gathering. Finally, behaviors of object agents include calling for help, being transferred, and participating in rescue actions. Based on behavior characteristics of each agent, interactions between agents in medical rescue force allocation systems during earthquakes include interactions between different agents, between different objects of the same agents, and between agents and the environment (Fig. 5.4). Force agents interact with

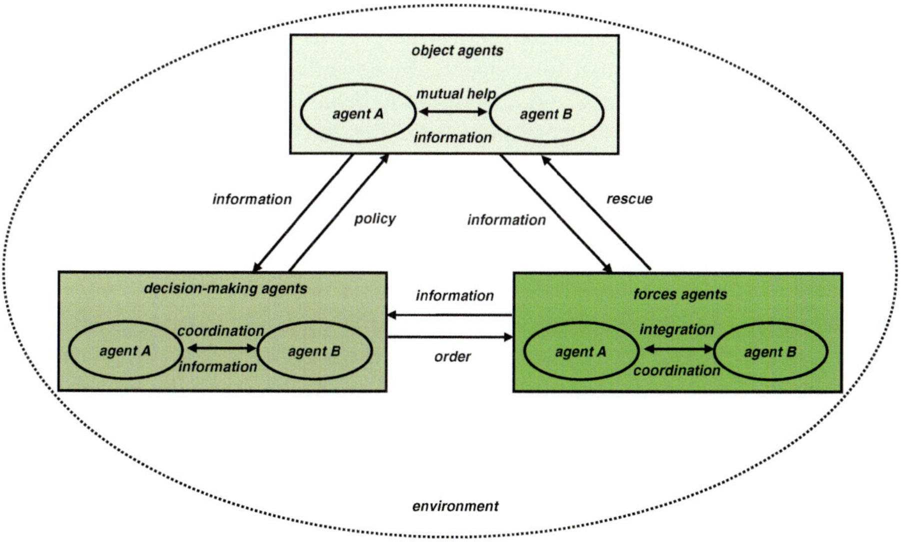

Fig. 5.4 Multi-agent interaction framework of medical rescue forces allocation during earthquakes

decision-making agents by transmitting treatment information on the sick and the wounded and information on health and epidemic prevention. Their medical treatment and epidemic prevention results directly affect behaviors of decision-making agents and change the properties and states of decision-making agents. The object agents conduct force mobility and allocation based on the information of the object agents and force agents and affect the force agents and object agents. Interactions between object agents and force agents result in changes in generating law of the sick and the wounded, affecting the efficiency of medical service actions, and thus causing property changes of decision-making agents. Between the object agents, there are interactions of mutual aid and exchanges of information. Between the force agents, there are interactions of combination and coordination. Finally, between the decision-making agents, there are interactions of coordination and information transfer. These three agents all exist under certain circumstances, and meanwhile, for each agent, it is also an environment for others, and through interactions and behavior changes, they can change the environment, properties, and states of other agents.

5.3.3.2 Multi-Agent Interaction Process of Medical Rescue Force Allocation During Earthquakes

Changes in the properties of object agents or a significant decrease in cumulative incidence will change the content and property of the decision-making agents, and the decision-making agents will send medical forces according to the current treatment situations, resulting in decision-making behaviors. This behavior changes the allocation quantity and properties of allocation forms, thereby resulting in corresponding behaviors. During this period, the key issue is to establish the relationship between the cumulative growth rate of the number of wounded individuals and the number of force agents. Meanwhile, there are changes in load properties of the force agents, and in addition to behavior changes that affect their own allocation, there are also interactions with other decision-making agents, which change the contents and mechanisms of the decision-making agents as well as the emergency medical service programs. At the same time, with the changes in behavior disciplines of agents, they will also cause changes in the other agents of the system. For example, the old rule of the object agents is "implementing treatment by a single medical team, and carry out treatment in the recent areas where the injured are focused," but if according to the new rules, "based on advanced technologies in the frontlines, there is a homogeneous concept of the front and rear treatments, and this strengthens the professional medical forces," the properties of the decision-making agents will also change. This will then act on the force agents, thus leading to property changes in the object agents. This is also a method for decision-making agents to continue learning and improve decision-making strategies and mechanisms through the process of interactions. As another example, interactions between the medical forces and epidemic prevention forces in force agents can affect not only the integration of "medicine, prevention, and recovery" in victims

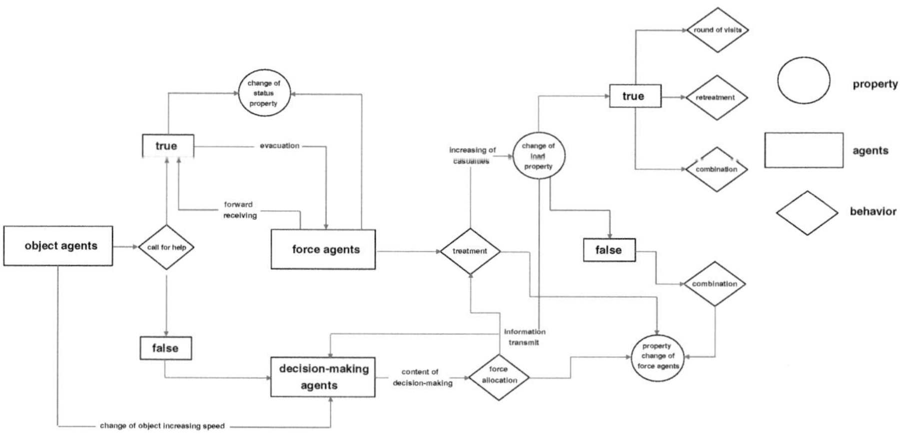

Fig. 5.5 Multi-agent interaction process of medical rescue force allocation during earthquakes

but also changes in environmental conditions. The rules of medical rescue force allocation in earthquake are manifestations of interactions between various agents. Through such interactions, the systems can realize the established goals and show their evolution processes (Fig. 5.5).

5.4 Analysis of Medical Rescue Forces Allocation Model in Earthquake

5.4.1 Systemic Simulation

Medical rescue force allocation during earthquakes shows three stages. The research group previously conducted empirical analyses of the medical rescue following the Wenchuan earthquake, finding that earthquake casualties were distributed across "two phases" (growth phase and steady phase) and that the utilization of emergency medical rescue forces (including force mobility and allocation) was divided into "three stages." Thus, emergency medical rescue after earthquakes showed the basic characteristics of "two phases and three stages," and based on this law, medical rescue in earthquake conducts organization command, utilization of forces, and organization management of task conversions (Fig. 5.6). Take Wenchuan earthquake as an example: the first phase of force utilization in emergency medical rescue following the earthquake occurred within 72 h after the earthquake, representing the emergency phase of medical rescue action. The second phase is from 72 h to 2 weeks after the earthquake, which is the effective stage for medical rescue actions. These two phases are the growth stages with regard to casualties. The third phase begins 2 weeks after the earthquake, and this is the maintenance phase of medical rescue actions and the stable stage with regard to casualties. In the emergency phase,

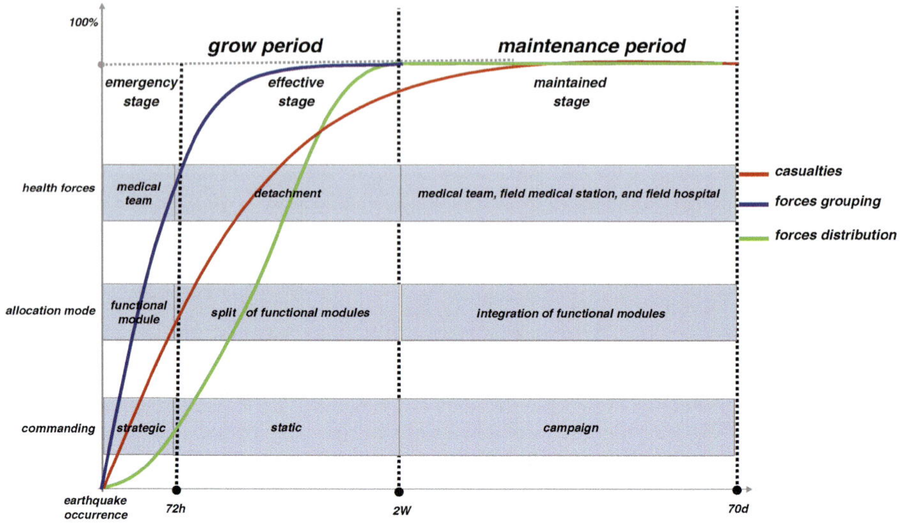

Fig. 5.6 Characteristics of "two phases and three stages" during medical rescue efforts following the Wenchuan earthquake

a large number of casualties occur, and rescue forces are mobilized in accordance with the function module, but rescue force allocation is disordered. In this stage, casualties continue to rise, and the main method of rescue force allocation is based on the split of function modules and splitting medical teams into small detachments to cover all hardest-hit areas. In the maintenance phase, casualties reach the saturation point, and the main method of rescue force allocation is integrating function modules of the five areas of responsibility and forming a responsible area module allocation system for medical teams, field clinics, and field hospitals. In each stage of the medical rescue following an earthquake, rescue force mobility and allocation each show different characteristics, and they are closely related to the utilization efficiency of medical rescue forces following an earthquake. Therefore, when analyzing the mobility and allocation of medical rescue forces after an earthquake, we can conduct analyses according to the features of the stage and consider the consistency of mobility and allocation of medical rescue forces simultaneously.

The first phase is the emergency stage. In this stage, a large number of casualties occur and rescue forces are mobilized in accordance with the function module; however, rescue force allocation is disordered. Medical rescue protections are mainly healthcare, first aid, and protecting victims. The second phase is the effective stage, in which casualties continue to rise, medical rescue command is mainly the tactical command of the squad, the main method of rescue forces allocation is based on the split of function modules, and medical teams are split into small detachments to cover all hardest-hit areas. Medical rescue protection turns into a combination of medical rescue, health and epidemic prevention, and mental relief. Medical rescue converts into emergency treatment and early treatment (damage control surgery),

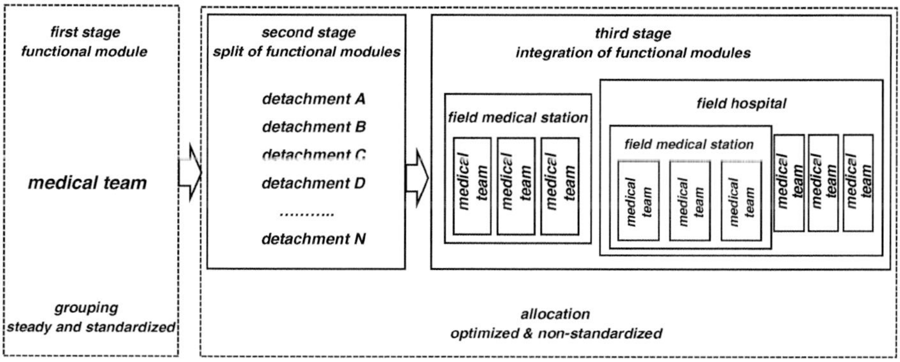

Fig. 5.7 Force mobility and allocation at each phase of medical rescue after the Wenchuan earthquake

and the protection objects change from victims to troops. The third phase is the maintenance stage, in which casualties reach a saturation point, a responsible command system is established in disaster areas, the main method of rescue forces allocation is integrating function modules of the five areas of responsibility, and a responsible module allocation system of medical teams, field clinics, and field hospitals is established (Fig. 5.7). Medical rescue turns into professional treatment (definitive treatment). Overall, medical rescue force mobility mainly involves the first and second phases, and the third phase does not involve mobilization of medical rescue forces. The second and third phases mainly adjust force allocation.

5.4.2 *Intervention*

5.4.2.1 The Peak of Casualties Appears in Advance, Which Suggests That the Efficiency Is Improving

Compared with the Wenchuan earthquake, the peak of casualties in the Yushu earthquake clearly appears earlier. The peak of casualties (calculated by 90 % of the cumulative percentage) appears 7 days in advance, and peak of sick and wounded individuals (calculated by 90 % of the cumulative percentage) appears 10 days in advance. Meanwhile, the reported death cumulative percentage and the reported casualty cumulative percentage within 72 h after the Yushu earthquake increased significantly. Gao Jianguo, who analyzed statistics regarding processes of earthquake information (casualties) released both domestically and abroad, suggested that the reported time of earthquake casualties is related with the total number of casualties, and the sooner the reported time of casualties approximates the total number of earthquake casualties, the stronger the rescue capability will be. By analyzing the time sequence of casualties in the Wenchuan and Yushu earthquakes, on the one hand, it was indicated that the "vacuum period" of medical rescue force allocation in Yushu earthquake was shortened, and the reported time of casualties in disaster areas was earlier than that in the Wenchuan earthquake; on the other hand, through the experiences of the Wenchuan earthquake, the effectiveness of medical rescue actions following the Yushu earthquake was significantly enhanced, and the efficiency of medical rescue force allocation improved. Deaths in the Tangshan earthquake accounted for 25.6 % of the total casualties, while in Wenchuan earthquake, this value was 19.3 %. Compared with the Wenchuan and Tangshan earthquakes, casualties in the Yushu earthquake decreased appreciably, and the percentage of casualties of all casualties decreased simultaneously, suggesting that the effectiveness of medical rescue following the Yushu earthquake improved significantly (Kang et al. 2012; Liu et al. 2012; Zhang et al. 2012).

5.4.2.2 Mobility and Allocation Have Good Consistency and the Integration of Decision-Making Is Continuous

Following the Wenchuan earthquake, medical rescue force allocation lagged behind, and within 72 h after the earthquake, among about 60 % of the strategic support forces that were mobilized, only 20 % were launched to conduct treatment in disaster areas. Compared with the rescue effort in Wenchuan, medical rescue force mobility and allocation in Yushu earthquake were almost synchronous, and this reduced inefficient losses by nearly 40 % within the first 72 h. Because of rapid force allocation and treatment, the cumulative growth time of the sick and wounded shortened, also reflecting the efficiency of actions following the Yushu earthquake. Twelve days after Wenchuan earthquake, the cumulative growth of the sick and the wounded accounted for 93.13 % of the total, while in the Yushu earthquake at this time, the cumulative growth of the sick and the wounded accounted for 99.61 % of the total. The consistency of medical rescue force mobility and allocation across the two earthquakes reflects the interaction among the object agents, force agents, and decision-making agents. Due to differences in the characteristic and laws of the object agents between the Wenchuan and Yushu earthquakes, the allocation times, methods, and properties of force agents in the Wenchuan earthquake are different from those in the Yushu earthquake.

The medical rescue forces in Wenchuan earthquake were allocated according to the "three-stage" type, mobilized within 72 h by function modules, function modules were split into squads from 72 h to 2 weeks and integrated into module system allocation after 2 weeks, and the medical rescue protection in the Yushu earthquake was mobilized and allocated according to the module system. From the beginning of the rescue actions, the module allocation system of the medical teams, epidemic prevention teams, and field shelter hospitals was formed, and medical treatment in Wenchuan was changed into an integration of medical treatment, epidemic prevention, and reconstruction. Further, the overall efficiency of medicine, epidemic prevention, and reconstruction was improved, and the force allocation also showed characteristics of the continuous integration of medicine, prevention, and recovery. Combined with the significance of the time sequence of casualties following the earthquake, it is thought that information on the object agents is transferred in advance, which promotes the contents and properties of the decision-making agents as well as the consistency of force allocation and transfer.

5.4.2.3 Adhere to Rapid, Flexible, and Scientific Allocation

It can be seen from the utilization of medical rescue forces following the Wenchuan and Yushu earthquakes, the utilization of forces should grasp the "three rapidness" stages, that is, the rapid medical rescue force mobility, rapid medical rescue force allocation, and rapid evacuation of the wounded. After large-scale disasters, the medical and health systems will be severely damaged in disaster areas, so the main medical rescue forces are the supporting force. This has been demonstrated in the Wenchuan and Yushu earthquakes, Hurricane Katrina, and the Haitian earthquake, among others. Therefore, the mobility and allocation of medical rescue forces must be rapid in order to achieve the target of "early and sufficient action, utilization of selected troops, and utilization of the nearest military forces." The healthcare system in disaster areas is unable to respond to a large number of treatment demands from the sick and wounded, and so casualties must be evacuated rapidly and safely, which is the key to reducing the morbidity and disability rates. Meanwhile, we must adhere to the "three successions," that is, medical rescue force mobility and actual allocation in disaster areas must be continuous, casualty evacuation and treatment must be continuous, and casualty evacuation across various levels must be continuous. After the disaster, whether the health forces mobilized to stricken areas are effectively allocated and whether they are consistent with the demands are the keys to the efficiency of force utilization. Therefore, we should ensure the continuity of force mobility and disaster allocation, mobilizing rapidly and allocating accurately, and improving the utilization efficiency of supporting forces. In the process of casualty evacuation, a variety of vehicles are often included, and the accompanied medical treatment in vehicles is the key to ensure safe evacuation. Among the evacuation levels, the transmission of casualty injury and medical care information is also extremely important. Therefore, it is necessary to load professional medical treatment equipment on the evacuation vehicles, allocate all professional staff, and conduct casualty information transmittance during the transfer period, thereby ensuring the continuity between evacuation and treatment and in evacuation across various levels.

During the two on-site studies, medical rescue commanders and medical rescue personnel all agreed that 24 h after the earthquake is the critical period of medical rescue, and within 8 h of the earthquake is before the critical period of "saving lives." Professional medical care personnel play the most critical role within 72 h after the earthquake, and they can conduct evacuations in succession after 72 h. The remaining medical rescue forces should make their visitation rounds as early as possible, and the specialist forces can be supplemented through rotation. This is also a result of evolution and learning with regard to medical rescue force allocation following earthquakes. In the Yushu earthquake, medical forces began retracement 9 days after the earthquake, and supporting forces of other provinces (except military field shelter hospitals) all completed retracement and construction 17 days after the earthquake (April 30th). Regional supporting forces also completed retracement,

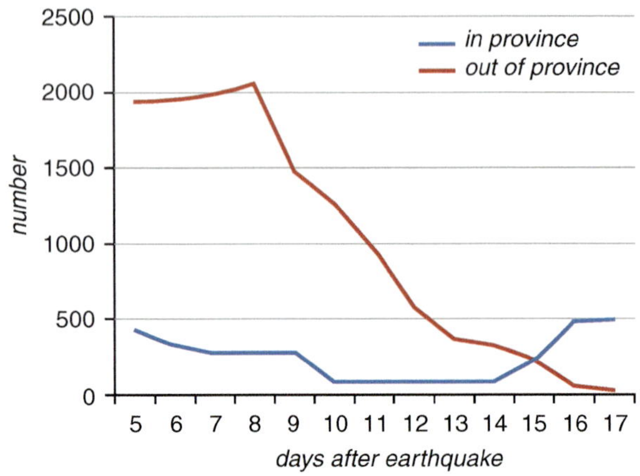

Fig. 5.8 Changes in medical forces participating in the Yushu earthquake after April 18, 2010

which mainly played the role of medical substitution during reconstruction in disaster areas (Fig. 5.8). Compared with the medical forces retreat after 70 days following the Wenchuan earthquake, force allocation decisions following the Yushu earthquake were more scientific and were made in accordance with the characteristic laws of the occurrence of the sick and wounded. The increase in epidemic prevention forces in the Yushu earthquake was designed to meet the needs of epidemic prevention in disaster areas and to suit the needs of plague foci in disaster areas. This was similar to the increase in epidemic prevention forces in the second phase of the Wenchuan earthquake, but in the Wenchuan earthquake, this problem was solved to some extent by converting medical teams into epidemic prevention forces, reflecting the principle of flexible allocation according to the needs of medical rescue forces.

5.5 Summary

According to the characteristics of medical rescue force allocation following earthquakes, we proposed some suggestions about medical rescue force construction and utilization following earthquakes.

5.5.1 Consistent with the Basic Principles of Utilization of Emergency Medical Rescue Forces, Realize the Modularization of Force Utilization During the Entire Process

Under emergency conditions, the utilization of emergency medical rescue forces should be based on emergency health needs and the intentions of emergency rescue command institutions. Further, they should consider the terrain and road conditions, epidemiology characteristics, and other medical geography to analyze the developmental trend of events and, based on this objective reality, adhere to the following principles. First, in accordance with the emergency conditions, the requirements of emergency medical rescue must be met. Emergency medical rescue forces should be beneficial to the on-site first aid of the sick and wounded, as well as facilitate rapid elimination and effective control of the consequences of events. Second, form an efficient emergency medical rescue system. Normally, such a system should be formed in accordance with different regions, points, lines, and planes, as well as the clustering allocation of different forces. This will allow for the combination of the local forces in the affected areas, regional supporting forces, and strategic supporting forces; the combination of regional allocation and linear allocation; the combination of prevention, treatment, and evacuation forces; and finally, the prevention of disjointed medical evacuation and health and epidemic prevention and avoidance of overlapping forces. Third, adapt to the objective conditions of roads and traffic. Rescue forces should be close to the main roads, have enough land and corresponding water, and be in close proximity to other rescue forces, thereby facilitating emergency medical rescue for the other rescue forces. Meanwhile, they should strive to avoid possible natural disasters or spreading locations, such as floods, landslides, and downwind direction of nuclear and chemical accidents. Emergency medical rescue force mobility must follow the function modules, the elements and types of service preparation should be well appointed, and the method of module allocation should be adopted throughout the entire process. Combined with different mission requirements and in accordance with module allocation requirements, treatment function modules should be established to adapt to different geographical, natural, and technical conditions. Furthermore, rescue forces should strengthen the construction of medical treatment function modules and the construction of structure standards, as well as promote the conversion of resources to security forces. Meanwhile, this requires improving types of functional element modules, which must be equipped with the necessary professional rescue modules, such as resources for obstetrics and gynecology, pediatrics, and psychology, thus realizing a multifunction professional module in addition to good mobility and portability.

5.5.2 *Using Strategic Regional and Local Forces Flexibly, Achieving Consistency in the "Three Stages" of Mobility and Allocation*

Strategic supporting forces are usually the "first" forces when emergency medical rescues are deployed following an earthquake, with characteristics of advanced technology and equipment and a high degree of standardization. Comparing between Wenchuan and Yushu, the strategic supporting forces were significantly improved, and the strategic supporting forces were superior to the other two rescue forces in both structural proportions and the technical level. The strategic supporting forces played an important role in first-line treatment in disaster areas, and the main advantage lies in their strong professional treatment capacity. Currently, there is a need to further enhance the mobility capacity of strategic supporting forces to allow for all-weather and all-around support for rapid mobility. As the supporting forces near the disaster areas, the regional supporting forces are important for early treatment and response, and the advantages of regional supporting forces in emergency medical rescue forces in the Yushu earthquake were mainly attributable to rapid mobility and allocation, as well as the ability to adapt to the high-altitude conditions. The local forces in disaster areas are mainly responsible for the emergency treatment after earthquakes and emergency treatment tasks. In the Yushu earthquake, the local emergency medical rescue forces were mainly mixed with supporting forces in the later period, which not only solved the language barrier issue faced by supporting forces but also improved the utilization efficiency of the local forces. In general, the utilization of strategic, regional, and local emergency medical rescue forces still lack a unified allocation principle and basis. In future earthquake emergency medical rescues, the utilization principles of emergency medical rescue forces should be established at all levels, the responsibilities and rescue needs of different levels of supporting forces should be clarified, strategic supporting forces should apply technical guidance and support, and regional supporting forces should conduct relevant technologic forces protection or corresponding supporting protection in the affected regions. All types of professional forces should be used collectively. The localization management in disaster areas (according to the areas of responsibility) and regional protection should be applied, and the scope of treatment technologies and the casualty evacuation system should be determined. Combined with the characteristics of the "two phases and three stages" of emergency medical rescue in earthquake, the utilization of emergency medical rescue forces should be in accordance with the characteristics of different periods for appropriate mobilization and allocation. Emergency rescue should fully consider the characteristics of the substantial medical needs of disaster areas, mobilizing rescue forces early, adequately, efficiently, and modularly. Force allocation should be rapid and forward, the module allocation system should be established throughout the entire process, a high degree of consistency between force mobility and allocation should be achieved, inefficient losses of forces utilization should be reduced, and the efficiency of emergency medical rescue should be reduced.

5.5.3 Emphasize Construction of Emergency Medical Rescue Forces Following Earthquakes and Allocate Professional Forces Rationally According to Demands

Trauma and crush injuries account for more than 80 % of injuries in earthquakes, significantly increasing the demand for professional surgical treatment. It is necessary to establish professional medical treatment forces and emphasize professional treatment. For example, the rapid response medical reinforcement teams of the US military have specially established trauma and emergency treatment rapid response reinforcement teams, which can use local equipment, resources, and portable medical kits for emergency medical treatment for the wounded, help determine the need for follow-up professional technologies and medical resources, and help develop a treatment transition plan to restore order and normality. Good professional treatment is crucial for the completion of earthquake emergency medical rescue. Therefore, to continually improve the establishment of national emergency medical rescue forces, the opportunity should be taken to establish earthquake emergency medical rescue professional teams, and the force unit should improve to the goal of being dedicated, structurally stable, and able to achieve rapid mobility. Earthquake emergency medical rescue professional teams should be established, and professional treatment experiences in emergency medicine and severe trauma treatment and methods should be accumulated through daily medical practices. Furthermore, it is necessary to conduct intensive daily training for the medical unit. For various kinds of personnel in medical teams, training must be conducted for on-site first aid for the sick and wounded, including ventilation, bleeding, bandaging, fixation transportation, and technical training on basic life support. This will allow members to skillfully use the corresponding tools and equipment, learn standard writing and transmission of injury tickets, registries, and simple medical record. Members of medical teams must be aware of the treatment of common diseases in earthquakes, such as the on-site first aid for crush syndrome. Meanwhile, consideration must be given to dealing with hypoxia syndrome in the highland plateau when conducting missions, handling heat stroke when operating at high temperatures, and dealing with frostbite when operating in cold seasons. Further, the professional forces should be emphasized with consideration to module allocation and utilization.

Professional forces should allocate according to demands. First, medical evacuation force allocation should be in accordance with on-site first aid and professional treatment and, if necessary, arrange early treatment stages. Based on localization management and requirements of regional protection, the protection regions must be divided uniformly and the scope of treatment technologies and the casualty evacuation system are determined. In unexpected events with a large number of casualties, the on-site emergency treatment forces often only include a range of first aid and emergency treatment technologies, such as simple lifesaving surgeries, emergency resuscitation for sustaining life, and simple debridement techniques. Once the wounded have maintained a stable condition, the nearest possible evacuation should be organized. Under emergency events with a large number of casualties, especially large disasters, public health command departments should allocate professional medical evacuation forces by railways, waterways, roads, and air and give priority to implement long-range evacuations by air. Second, the health and epidemic prevention forces should be allocated based on principles of the combination of primary and professional epidemic prevention forces and the combination of mobilized forces and regional forces. National, local, and military health administrative departments should organize epidemic prevention and control as well as health supervision in accordance with conditions; arrange forces in affected areas to conduct health epidemiological surveys, evaluation, and health inspection; send on-site disposal forces; and take effective preventative and control measures to prevent secondary or derivative public health emergencies caused by various types of emergencies. The responsibilities and rescue needs of different levels of supporting forces must be clarified, with the strategic supporting forces implementing technical guidance and supports and regional supporting forces conducting relevant technological force protection or corresponding supporting protection in the regions. Regional epidemic prevention forces for emergencies should implement corresponding on-site disposals.

References

Abolghasemi H, Poorheidari G, Mehrabi A, Foroutan G. Iranian military forces in the Bam earthquake. Military Med. 2005;170(10):859–61.

Amundson D, Lane D, Ferrara E. Operation Aftershock: the US military disaster response to the Yogyakarta earthquake May through June 2006. Military Med. 2008;173(3):236–40.

Bilham R. Lessons from the Haiti earthquake. Nature. 2010;463(7283):878–9.

Chen Z, Shen J, Kang J X, et al. Emergency medical rescue after major earthquakes: lessons from the Wenchuan earthquake [J]. Chin J Evid-Based Med. 2012;12(4):383–92.

Jiang J, You-Ping LI, Lin Huang X, Bing LI, Lin SU, Ke Zhong S, Hu Shi C, Ming-Xu LI, Shan J. Lessons learnt from Wenchuan earthquake: performance evaluation for treatment of critical injuries in extremely-hit areas after great earthquake. Chinese J Evid-Based Med. 2012;12(5): 504–11.

Jiang J, Li Y P, Wang M Y, et al. Comparison of Yushu earthquake and Wenchuan earthquake in medical rescue [J]. China J Evid Based Med. 2010;10:550–54.

Kang P, Zhang L, Liang W, Zhu Z, Liu Y, Xu L, Yang H. Medical evacuation management and clinical characteristics of 3,255 inpatients after the 2010 Yushu earthquake in China. J Trauma-Injury Infect Crit Care. 2012;72(6):1626–33.

Liu X, Zhang L L, Liu Y, et al. Comparative analysis on the characteristics of casualties medical evacuation in Wenchuan and Yushu earthquakes [J]. Chin J Evid-Based Med. 2012;12: 512–15.

Merin O, Ash N, Levy G, et al. The Israeli field hospital in Haiti—ethical dilemmas in early disaster response [J]. New England Journal of Medicine. 2010;362(11):e38.

Xiao-Ming LI. Organization and command of medical rescue in Yushu earthquake. Hosp Admin J Chinese Peoples Liber Army. 2010 (8):701–703.

Yuan L, Xu L, Peng K, Zeng-hong Z, Xing-biao S, Zhi-peng L, Lu-lu Z. Strategic supporting forces grouping in emergency medical relief of Yushu earthquake. Hosp Admin J Chinese Peoples Liber Army. 2011;18(4):384–85.

Yuan L, Zhang Y, Yang H, Xu L. Characteristics of military health forces use in earthquake medical rescue. Chinese J Evid-Based Med. 2014;14(4):373–5.

Zhang L, Liu X, Zhang Y, Liu Y. Medical support in Wenchuan earthquake relief: characteristics and reflections. Hosp Admin J Chinese Peoples Liber Army. 2008;15(11):1014–16.

Zhang L, Xu L, Li Y, Liu Y, Liu Z, Lin J, Shen J, Tang X, Zhang Y, Liang W. Emergency medical rescue efforts after a major earthquake: lessons from the 2008 Wenchuan earthquake. Lancet. 2012;379(9818):853–61.

Zhang L, Liu Y, Xu L, Zhang Y. Rescue efforts management and characteristics of casualties of the Wenchuan earthquake in China. Emerg Med J. 2011;28(7):618–22.

Chapter 6
Modeling the Organization and Command of Earthquake Rescue Forces

Wei An and Lulu Zhang

Abstract In recent years, China has suffered major natural disasters, resulting in huge losses. At the same time, with experience in disasters, we have formed an emergency management system of military and civilian integration, with military and police collaboration and civilian involvement in extensive mobilization of domestic forces. The Yushu earthquake medical rescue mission showed the response of different departments of both military and civilians and their cooperative command mechanism when facing complex missions. We divided all units in the rescue mission into three types of agents: R-agents, P-agents, and matchmakers. We then summarized the coordination mechanism as "two-level four-unit" Joint Assembly. Using a multi-agent system, NK model, and MATLAB software, our purpose is to present a behavioral modeling for some applications using autonomous agents in real environments (geographical regions) and show that this can be a useful approach for simulation of complex systems (military conflicts, urban and environmental phenomena, etc.).

6.1 Introduction

6.1.1 Background

In recent years, China has suffered major natural disasters, resulting in substantial losses. At the same time, with experience in disasters, we have formed an emergency management system with military and civilian integration, military and police collaboration, civilian involvement in extensive mobilization of domestic forces,

W. An
Department of Diving Medicine, Naval Medical Research Institute, Shanghai 200433, China

L. Zhang (✉)
Department of Military Health Service, College of Military Health Service, Second Military Medical University, Shanghai, China
e-mail: zllrmit@aliyun.com

© Springer Science+Business Media Dordrecht 2016

L. Zhang (ed.), *Modeling the Injury Flow and Treatment after Major Earthquakes*, DOI 10.1007/978-94-017-7527-4_6

emergency management in the military, and civilian-integrated roads with Chinese characteristics, showing a trend of diversification (Zhang et al. 2011; Zhang et al. 2012; Zhu 2009). This study was conducted on the national conditions of our country that make it prone to natural disasters, Yushu earthquake medical relief, the trend of diversification in response to a variety of security threats, and accomplishment of diverse military mission capability requirements to carry out the collaborative command mechanism.

Many important and useful applications for software agents require multiple agents on a network that communicate with each other (Wagner 2002; Davidson et al. 2002). Such agents must find each other and perform a useful joint computation without having to know about every other such agent in the network (Pastor 2001). For example, this paper describes a matchmaker system, designed to find people with similar interests and introduce them to each other. The matchmaker is designed to introduce everyone, unlike conventional Internet media, which only allow those who take the time to speak in public to be known (Bilham 2010). This paper details how the agents that comprise the matchmaking system can function in a decentralized fashion, yet group themselves into clusters which reflect their users' interests; these clusters are then used to make introductions or allow users to send messages to others who share their interests.

6.1.2 Concepts and Theories

Synergy refers to the coordination of two or more than two different resources or individuals to complete the process of a goal or concerted ability. This synergy enhances the resources or individuals involved, and coherence toward a common positive direction is collaborative (Abolghasemi et al. 2005). Collaborative study on a given topic forms coordination theory. Synergetic theory is found on the base of system theory, information theory, cybernetics, and mutation theory, as well as part of the theory of dissipative structure, and by analyzing different fields on the method of combining statistics and dynamics, the theory establishes the mathematical model and a complete set of processing schemes on the transition of micro to macro as well as describes common rules from disorder to order in various kinds of system and the phenomenon (Depew et al. 1996).

The disaster medical rescue system is a complex, large, and open system consisting of human, technology, and material support (Hu 2012; Jennings 1995). There are several elements to such a system, where each element is a nested set of multiple secondary elements with internal nonlinear characteristics (Li et al. 2011; Ligtenberg et al. 2004). The exchange of material and information between the system environment and the external world is in line with the research scope of synergetic systems. Systems with information on every little change in the external environment for internal work are adjusted accordingly. At the same time, different departments in the system connect and interact mutually, and they have their own differences also.

If no disasters happen, there is no internal contact in the system, and each subsystem works independently, and this makes the disaster medical rescue system disordered (Li et al. 2011; Ligtenberg et al. 2004). If some disaster happened, the system would run under the guidance of collaborative, and interactions such as information sharing and communication would happen between subsystems; then the system would gradually run from disorder to order.

6.1.3 Objective and Significance

Our purpose was to present behavioral modeling for some applications using autonomous agents in real environments (geographical regions) and show that this can be a useful approach for the simulation of complex systems (military conflicts, urban and environmental phenomena, etc.).

This section presents an investigation of command and control during multi-agency operations; the purpose of this study was to elaborate on known themes associated with multi-agency emergency response through a study of the successful combined military and civilian units from the Yushu earthquake in April 2009. This case study demonstrates that effective coordination during major emergencies requires the development of a deeper, shared understanding of the incident and a high level of trust between responding organizations, both of which require effort to achieve and are difficult to support with current communications systems (Hosseini and Vaz 2005). Adoption of a socio-technical systems approach during the development process may enable future communications systems to support these important social processes.

Operations other than war are a real test of the joint military–civilian operations and provide a practical platform for military and civilian forms of collaboration for the new era of innovation (Amundson 2008). The basis of this research is collaborative theory, complex adaptive systems theory, multi-agent systems theory, and disaster medical rescue theory (Montano et al. 2008; Park and Sugumaran 2005). To make this research, we introduced analytic hierarchy process, gray relational analysis, Delphi, expert survey, consulting method, and other methods. To get more information on units which took part in the earthquake medical relief operations, we conducted a field investigation and a questionnaire survey in Yushu in Qinghai Province. The survey was based on the summary of data and expert advice on collaborative command of units under the context of nonwar military operations such as disaster medical rescue (Auerbach et al. 2010; Devi 2010). Then we could define the main attributes, rules of collaborative command, and the trend of diversification of operations other than war and improve the efficiency and effectiveness of collaborative command. By constructing mathematical models in simulation software, we could describe the abstraction mechanism and simulate the complex process of collaborative command. This allowed us to explore a variety of factors and provided new tools and methods for relevant theory.

6.2 Data Resource Used in the Model

6.2.1 Utilization of the Current Data Resource

We searched "multi-agent," "collaborative command," "collaborative control," "interagency coordination," "collaborative work," "negotiation and cooperation," "cooperation based," "group consensus," and "operation other than war" from journal databases such as Elsevier, Springer, and BMJ. We obtained more than 200 articles, 30 theses. And we got 7 reports from www.worldcat.org as well.

6.2.2 Data Source from Field Survey

To construct our field survey, our research group went to Yushu in December 2011 and obtained files including the following:

1. 50 briefings on duties from the Ministry of Health, 47 summaries, and 87 other documents
2. Chronicles of medical rescue events in earthquake relief work from the Ministry of Health
3. 49 messages on duties of medical rescue in the Yushu earthquake relief mission from the Health Department of Qinghai Province and more than 120 relevant reports
4. Information from 114 medical teams
5. Rescue actions within 72 h after the earthquake
6. Information about evacuation of the sick and wounded during the earthquake
7. Other files, including 14 expert interviews, 13 symposium records, and 69 expert questionnaires

6.2.3 Collection of Documents

We sent 90 questionnaires to the military units that had taken part in the rescue actions, and 76 questionnaires were returned.

6.3 Modeling the Organization and Command of Multi-agents

6.3.1 Definition of Earthquake Medical Rescue Force and Collaborative Analysis

More than 5000 medical staff took part in the Yushu rescue mission. Initially, the medical teams were mostly from the territorial medical system and were led by the

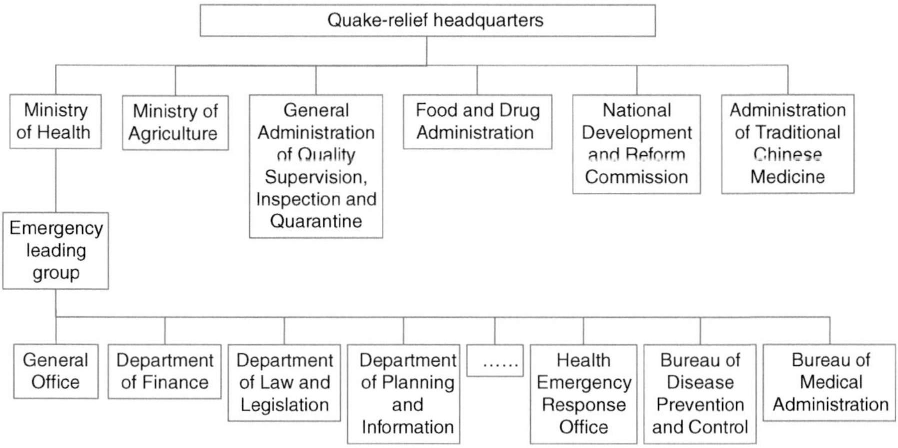

Fig. 6.1 Relationships among command agents

Ministry of Health, Department of Health of Qinghai Province, and the Bureau of Health of territorial cities. The subordinate relations were not very complex.

Later in the mission, more rescue teams from other provinces and from the army joined in, and the number of teams increased to 114, including 45 from Qinghai Province; 48 from Sichuan, Gansu, Shaanxi, and other provinces; and 21 from the army.

The State Council set up a quake-relief headquarters, which included the National Development and Reform Commission, Ministry of Agriculture, General Administration of Quality Supervision, Inspection and Quarantine, Food and Drug Administration, Ministry of Health, and Administration of Traditional Chinese Medicine.

The Ministry of Health set up an emergency leading group, including General Office, Department of Finance, Department of Law and Legislation, Department of Planning and Information, Department of Healthcare Reform, Health Emergency Response Office, Bureau of Disease Prevention and Control, Bureau of Medical Administration, Department of Primary Health, Department of Maternal and Child Health, Department of Food Safety Standards, Risk Surveillance and Assessment, Bureau of Inspection and Supervision, Department of Community Family Planning, Department of Family Development, and so on (Fig. 6.1).

The four units—Ministry of Health, Health Department of Qinghai Province, Health Department of General Logistics Department (GLD), and the Health Department of Lanzhou Military Region—constituted the command union for all rescue teams, and each rescue team had its own superior. The diverse characteristics are shown in Fig. 6.2.

6.3.1.1 Attributes of Medical Rescue Agents

Every team will be involved in the rescue operation as an agent, and its properties include basic attributes, working properties, and structural characteristics. Basic attributes refer to the nature and scope of duties. Working properties refer to

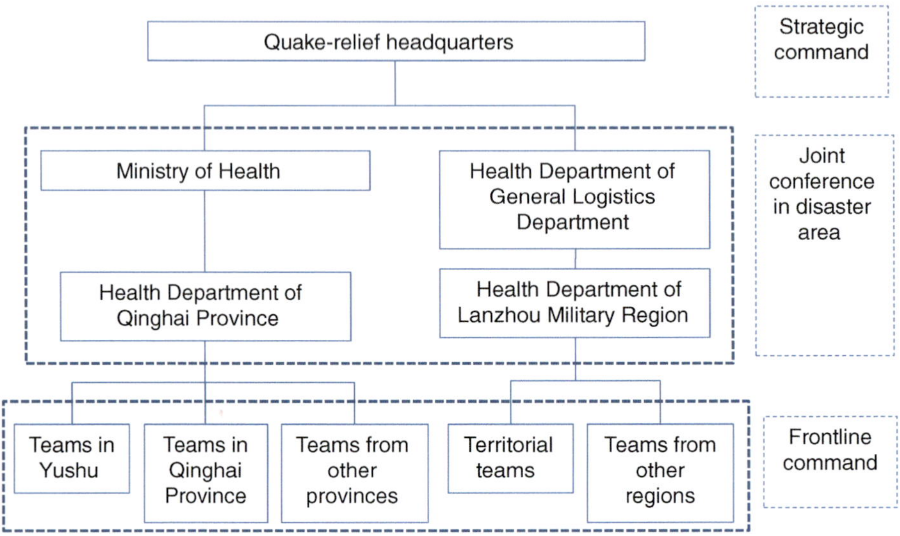

Fig. 6.2 Command agents in the Yushu rescue mission

manpower structure, location, relief scope, the rescue ability, work time, effort, and so on (Chen and Lee 2003). Structural characteristics refer to the subordinate relations, command hierarchy, and so on.

6.3.1.2 Attributes of Disaster Rescue Command Agents

The command agents in the earthquake rescue were all in the leadership of the quake-relief headquarters of the State Council and were made up from departments such as National Development and Reform Commission, Ministry of Agriculture, General Administration of Quality Supervision, Inspection and Quarantine, Food and Drug Administration, Ministry of Health, and the Administration of Traditional Chinese Medicine. Their duties and divisions are as follows:

(a) Ministry of Health:
Comprehensive coordination and daily routine work; contact information; collect and report the work; oversee work meeting conference organization and important work; overall national disaster relief medical treatment and healthcare power, health and epidemic prevention, and health supervision work, including medical treatment and transport of the wounded; send medical teams and experts to guide and support the disaster area in medical treatment and epidemic prevention and control to ensure the safety of the drinking water and food in the disaster area; provide guidance to the medical units and medical supplies, external publicity, information releasing, disease prevention knowledge propaganda, risk communication, and so forth
(b) National Development and Reform Commission
Health and epidemic prevention materials for seismic disaster relief emergency security work and coordination; act according to the requirements of the health

and epidemic prevention, and coordinate related departments to administer drugs, medical devices, and other key supplies, as well as address transportation, security aseismatic health, and epidemic prevention needs

(c) Ministry of Agriculture
Animal husbandry and veterinary work; collect, sort, and report earthquake relief anti-epidemic work information as needed and carry out instructions on death of livestock disinfection and disposal, animal epidemic monitoring, disease prevention, and control and quarantine supervision measures

(d) General Administration of Quality Supervision, Inspection, and Quarantine:
Inspection and quarantine work for the imported special reagents, equipment that was much needed.

(e) Food and Drug Administration:
Food safety, production, circulation, use, supervision, and management of medical apparatus and instruments and medicines required in emergency relief and quality of supervision and management of the donated medicine, medical apparatus and instruments (Domres et al. 2000); examination and approval of imported drugs and medical equipment to ensure the quality of drugs and medical appliances

(f) Administration of traditional Chinese medicine:
Select teams and traditional medicine expert guidance in the disaster areas to carry out the use of traditional medicine to treat patients and conduct disease prevention work.

(g) Health Department of GLD:
Organize relevant military health technical personnel and strength to guide and support territorial medical treatment and prevent disaster relief work.

(h) Logistics Department of People's Armed Police:
Organization of armed police forces to participate in earthquake relief and conduct medical treatment, military health and epidemic prevention, mental health services, and so on; to guide and support territorials in medical treatment, relief, epidemic prevention, and so forth.

6.3.1.3 Command in Medical System

The National Ministry of Health established the Ministry of Health emergency leading group for the Yushu earthquake in Qinghai Province through general information; medical treatment, prevention, and management of health; food and drinking water safety; logistics group; news propaganda team/group; and international cooperation in front of the working group.

(a) General information office:
Responsible for information contacting, collecting, and reporting, general coordination and routine work, organizing meetings and allocating important work, and other works

(b) Medical rescue group
Responsible for guiding and organizing medical treatment of the wounded as well as transport work, allocation of health resources, developing related therapeutic plans, and selecting medical teams

(c) Disease prevention and control group
Responsible for disaster relief disease prevention and control work, coordination, epidemic monitoring reports, environmental emergencies, vaccine immunization, and so on
(d) Food and water security group
Responsible for coordinating and guiding the disaster areas with regard to food safety, safety of drinking water, food and drinking water, security event monitoring, reporting, and disposal work and helps in guiding rescuers with regard to occupational protection
(e) Publicity and information group
The earthquake relief work is responsible for health system propaganda as well as health education and risk communication.
(f) Materials support group
Responsible for coordinating the implementation of disaster relief funds, relief material mixing, and unified management
(g) International group
Responsible for corresponding with the World Health Organization and other international organizations, in addition to national health departments of Hong Kong, Macao, and Taiwan
(h) Coordination group:
Responsible for guiding and assisting territorial medical rescue work and the disaster relief medical rescue team to coordinate the work ahead

6.3.2 Multi-agent Earthquake Medical Rescue Model

6.3.2.1 NK Model

In this rescue action, there are four command organizations: Ministry of Health, Health Department of Qinghai Province, Health Department of GLD, and Health Department of Lanzhou Military region, in addition to 114 medical teams from many provinces and the army. Thus, there are 118 agents in all (Table 6.1).

Table 6.1 Agents in the Yushu rescue mission

Type	Membership	Amounts
Command	Ministry of Health	1
	Health Department of GLD	1
	Health Department of Qinghai Province	1
	Health Department of Lanzhou Military Region	1
Rescue	Territorial teams	45
	Other provinces	48
	Territorial military region	8
	Other military regions	13
Total		118

The performance measure is as follows:

$$f = \frac{1}{118}\sum_{i=1}^{118} fi$$

For convenient description and analysis, according to the attribute of the rescue forces and the subordinate relations, 114 rescue teams were classified as territorial, with other provinces and cities to support the territorial health power strength, territorial military strength, and troops backed by four types of other support powers. There were four main behavioral bodies combined with four main command bodies, for a total of eight main bodies (Weinberger 1991; Cavalcante et al. 2012). The relationship between different agents is shown above.

For this NK model, $N = 8$, and the performance measure is as follows:

$$f = \frac{1}{8}\sum_{i=1}^{8} fi$$

In this model, contacts between the Ministry of Health and Health Department of GLD, between the Health Department of Qinghai Province and Health Department of Lanzhou Military Region, and among all rescue teams were lateral. Contacts between the Ministry of Health and Health Department of Qinghai Province and between Health Department of GLD and Health Department of Lanzhou Military Region were vertical integration. There was also vertical integration between command agents and rescue teams (Fig. 6.3).

6.3.2.2 Structure Matrix of Multi-agents

To take part in the rescue operation at various levels and of the main body of the function properties and behavioral characteristics, collaborative behavior between

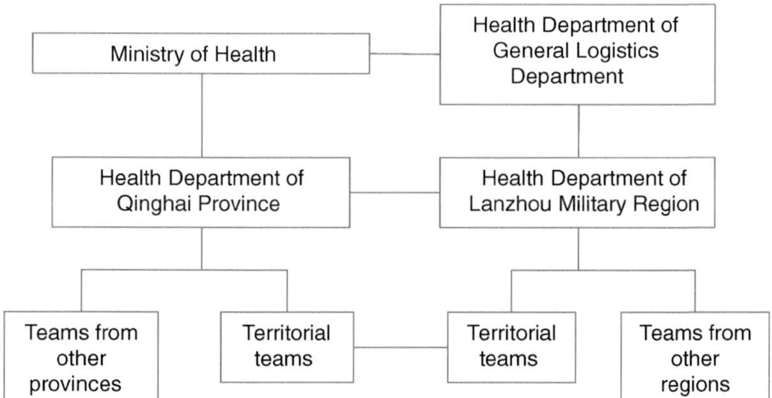

Fig. 6.3 Relationships among agents in Yushu

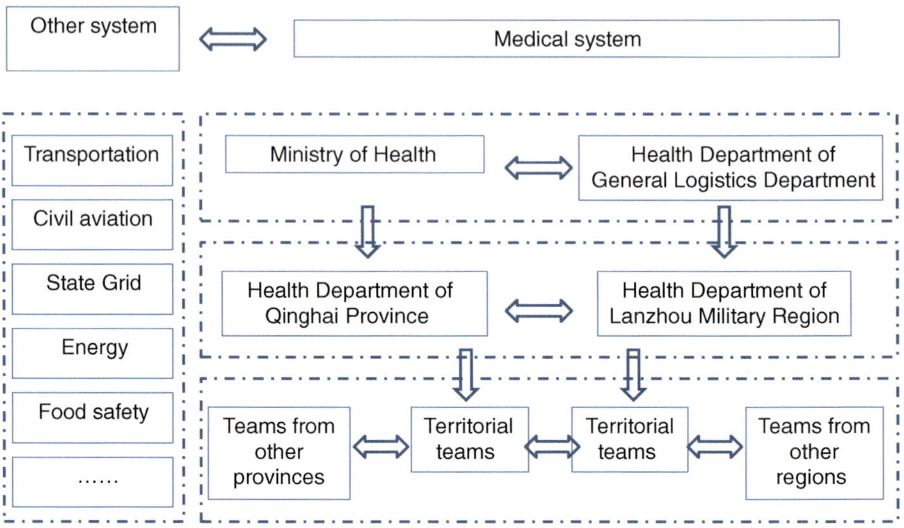

Fig. 6.4 Synergy relationships

the main body can be divided into three types: one is the system internal transverse integration synergy; the second is the coordination of the internal longitudinal command system; and the third is the system communication coordination with other external systems (Fig. 6.4).

1. Horizontal integration synergy
   Horizontal integration synergy is the most extensive coordination among different parts of the inner system (Baker 2007). Each main division of labor cooperation engages in information sharing and focuses on all aspects of knowledge, strength, and resources, forming the following resultant force:

   Synergy between the Ministry of Health and Health Department of GLD, synergy between Health Department of Qinghai Province and Health Department of Lanzhou Military Region, synergy between civil medical teams and military medical teams, synergy between territorial military rescue units and rescue units from other military regions. and synergy between territorial civil rescue units and rescue units from other provinces
2. Longitudinal integration synergy
   Longitudinal decentralization coordination refers to the subsystem of synergy, tasks detailed again after distribution within the subsystem, division of labor, cooperation, and coordination as follows:

   Synergy between Health Department of GLD and Health Department of Lanzhou Military Region, between the Health Department of Lanzhou Military Region and territorial military rescue units, between the Ministry of Health and Health Department of Qinghai Province, and between Health Department of Qinghai Province and territorial civil medical rescue teams
3. Synergy between system and the external world
   The external world mainly refers to the health system and railway, civil aviation, transportation, agriculture, and coordination between territorial government

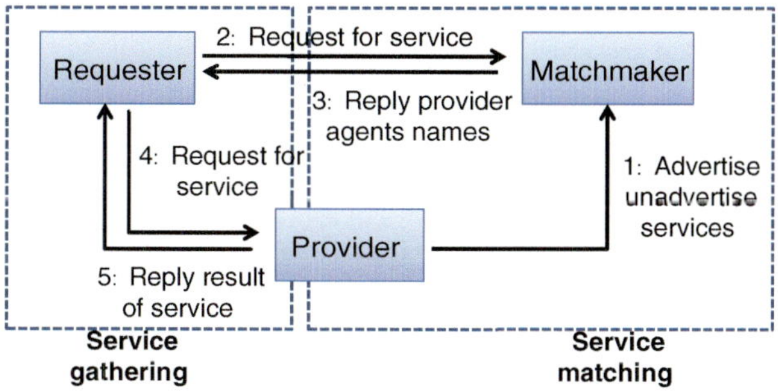

Fig. 6.5 Mode of action of the matchmaker model

Table 6.2 Attribution and actions of agents

Agent	Superior	Role	Function
Territorial civil teams	Health Department in Qinghai Province	R-agent	Sending requests to the superior for help
Territorial military teams	Territorial military region	P-agent	Providing help according to the emergency response plan
Other civil teams	Health departments of other provinces	P-agent	Providing help according to the order from superior
Other military teams	Other military regions	P-agent	Providing help according to the order from superior

and other units. In view of the different task types and content, the collaborative object also differs.

Thus, synergy occurred between the medical system and the railway, civil aviation, transportation, agriculture, and other departments.

6.3.2.3 Coordination Models Based on Matchmaker

In this rescue mission, the top matchmaker is the quake-relief headquarters, and then the matchmaker in medical system is the "two-level four-unit" Joint Assembly, which is made up of four command agents from the army and civilian population. Rescue teams in Qinghai Province are R-agents here, and rescue teams from other provinces and the army are P-agents (Fig. 6.5).

When rescue teams in Qinghai Province could not finish the rescue missions alone, they sent requests for help, and rescue teams from other provinces and other regions provided help. The quake-relief headquarters took the role of matchmaker, and the relationships are shown below (Table 6.2).

Besides, P-agents and R-agents in the system are relative. For example, rescue teams from Lanzhou military region are P-agents to the teams in Yushu, but to the teams from other provinces, they are R-agents (Table 6.3).

To the medical system, all units in the rescue mission can be divided into four categories, namely, territorial civil teams, territorial military teams, teams from other provinces, and teams from other military region. Their relationships are shown below (Fig. 6.6).

Table 6.3 Influences and role models among agents

Agents	Influence to themselves	Influence to other agents
Territorial civil teams	Manpower and materials loss, cannot finish the rescue mission	Get help and provide information to other agents
Territorial military teams	Short distance, but limited manpower and materials	Provide information to other agents
Other civil teams	Long distance, less information, and fewer goods and materials	Provide help to territorial medical units and require support for goods and materials
Other military teams	Long distance, less information, and less goods and materials	Provide help to territorial medical units and require support for goods and materials

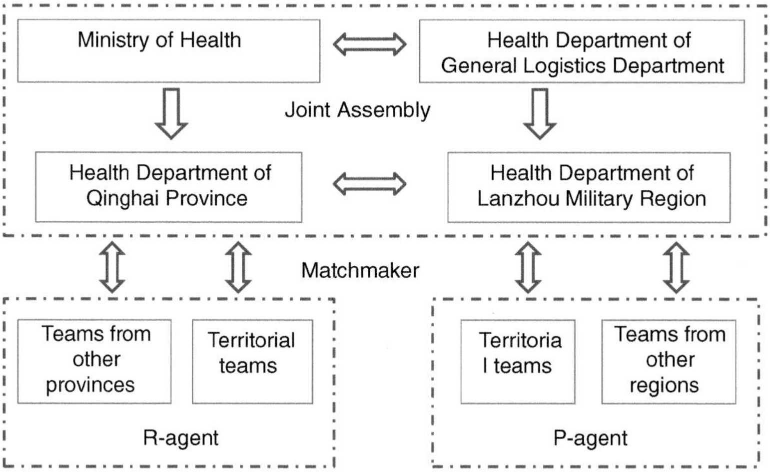

Fig. 6.6 Matchmaker model of the medical system for Yushu earthquake rescue

Synergy refers to a set of main bodies joined together through a series of activities of mutual cooperation. In the process of disaster relief, the cooperation between departments to deal with the effects of disasters is a common consensus, but the specific coordination mechanism and the effect of synergy mechanisms on dealing with disaster relief has been insufficiently researched. We defined three kinds of synergy mechanisms in this article (Table 6.4).

The synergy mechanism in Yushu is strong coordination because the "two-level four-unit" Joint Assembly played the role of matchmaker (Fig. 6.7).

6.3.2.4 Synergy Matrix in Yushu

This study gives priority to medical rescue, but the diversity of earthquake relief operations determines the complexity of the subject, in addition to the health system, also including transportation, railway, civil aviation, agriculture, and other

Table 6.4 Different kinds of synergy mechanisms

Type	Characteristic	Mode	Expression
No coordination	No contact or cooperation among agents	Do not send requests	No connections among agents
Weak coordination	Simple form of coordination	Sending requests to other agents directly and waiting for response	Sending requests to other agents one by one and waiting for a response for a long time
Strong coordination	Have a matchmaker	All requests and responses are checked by the matchmaker	Quick response

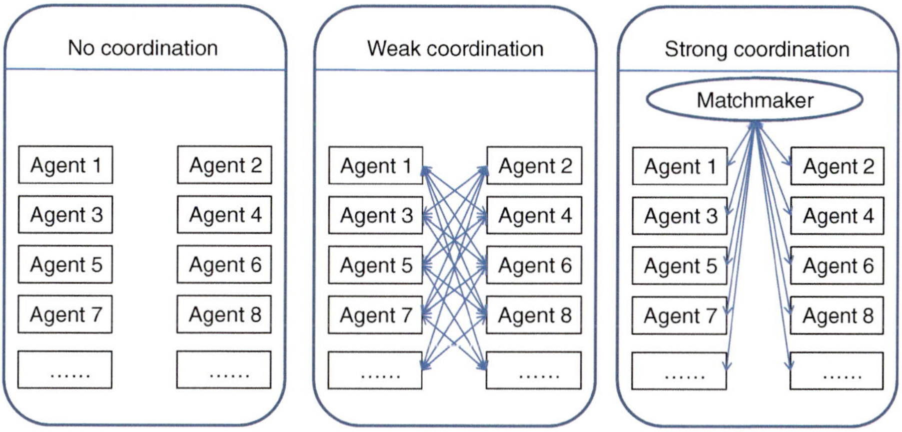

Fig. 6.7 Comparison of different synergy mechanisms (Yi et al. 2010)

departments and territorial governments at all levels. However, not all of the tasks of the collaborative process require the participation of various departments, according to the results of questionnaire survey and expert advice. Different types of rescue missions require different degrees of participation across departments (Lai and Coghill 1992). We then took transport of the transport and anti-epidemic to provide examples.

6.3.2.5 Matrix for Transport of the Wounded Work

During transport of the wounded, the military and territorial medical teams are involved in power, and the transportation, railway, and civil aviation departments are responsible for providing transport capacity as well as coordination with the city accepting the wounded individuals and provincial governments to participate in Yushu prefecture government. The collaborative relationship between different subjects is presented in the following table (Table 6.5).

Table 6.5 Synergy among departments when transporting the wounded

	Medical system				Transportation	Railway	Civil aviation	Agriculture	Food safety	Territorial government
	Territorial civil	External civil	Territorial military	External military						
Territorial civil	●	●	●	●	●					
External civil	●	●	●	●		●				
Territorial military	●	●	●	●	●					
External military	●	●	●	●	●	●	●			●
Transportation	●		●	●	●					
Railway		●		●		●				
Civil aviation				●			●			
Agriculture								●		
Food safety									●	
Territorial government				●						●

The matrix is as follows:

$$
\begin{bmatrix}
1 & 1 & 1 & 1 & & & & & & \\
1 & 1 & 1 & 1 & & 1 & & & & \\
1 & 1 & 1 & 1 & 1 & & & & & \\
1 & 1 & 1 & 1 & 1 & 1 & 1 & & & 1 \\
1 & & 1 & 1 & 1 & & & & & \\
 & 1 & & 1 & & 1 & & & & \\
 & & & 1 & & & 1 & & & \\
 & & & & & & & 1 & & \\
 & & & & & & & & 1 & \\
 & & & 1 & & & & & & 1
\end{bmatrix}
$$

6.3.2.7 Matrix for Epidemic Prevention

When epidemic prevention work is being conducted, army and territorial health epidemic prevention are involved in a team. In addition to the agriculture department being responsible for providing assistance, the transport department is responsible for health and epidemic prevention work requiring special equipment and transport vehicles. The territorial government is responsible for relevant publicity and education, populace mobilization, and other management and coordination responsibilities. The collaborative relationships between different subjects are presented below (Table 6.6).

The influence matrix is as follows:

$$
\begin{bmatrix}
1 & 1 & 1 & & & & & & \\
1 & 1 & 1 & 1 & 1 & & 1 & & 1 \\
1 & 1 & 1 & 1 & & & 1 & & 1 \\
1 & 1 & 1 & 1 & 1 & & 1 & & 1 \\
1 & & 1 & 1 & 1 & & & & \\
 & & & 1 & 1 & & & & \\
 & & & 1 & & 1 & & & \\
1 & 1 & 1 & 1 & & & 1 & & 1 \\
 & & & & & & & 1 & \\
1 & 1 & 1 & 1 & & & 1 & & 1
\end{bmatrix}
$$

The interactive work occurred mostly in the medical system, but also between the medical system and other systems when facing some kind of mission. When the mission was finished, the interactive work concluded. When dealing with different missions, parameter N is fixed, and parameter K varied.

6.3.2.8 Influence Matrix in Yushu

In Yushu, there are four command units and 114 rescue teams, and we can divide the 114 rescue teams into four categories, and each category represents an agent. Thus, there are four command agents and four rescue agents (Table 6.7).

Table 6.6 Synergy among departments in epidemic prevention

	Medical system									
	Territorial civil	External civil	Territorial military	External military	Transportation	Railway	Civil aviation	Agriculture	Food safety	Territorial government
Territorial civil	●	●	●	●				●		●
External civil	●	●	●	●				●		●
Territorial military	●	●	●	●				●		●
External military	●	●	●	●	●	●		●		●
Transportation				●	●					
Railway				●		●				
Civil aviation							●			
Agriculture	●	●	●	●				●		●
Food safety									●	
Territorial government	●	●	●	●				●		●

Table 6.7 Connections among rescue units

	Territorial civil rescue teams	Territorial military rescue teams	Other civil units	Other military units	Health Department in Qinghai	Health Department in Lanzhou Military Region	Ministry of Health	Health Department of GLD
Territorial civil rescue teams	●	●	●	●				
Territorial military rescue teams	●	●	●	●				
Other civil units	●	●	●	●				
Other military units	●	●	●	●				
Health Department in Qinghai	●	●	●	●	●			
Health Department in Lanzhou Military Region	●	●	●	●	●	●		
Ministry of Health	●	●	●	●	●	●	●	●
Health Department of GLD	●	●	●	●	●	●	●	●

The command agent can affect all the other rescue units, but the rescue teams only affect themselves, and then their relationship can be converted to a matrix as follows:

$$\begin{bmatrix} 1 & 1 & 1 & 1 & & & & \\ 1 & 1 & 1 & 1 & & & & \\ 1 & 1 & 1 & 1 & & & & \\ 1 & 1 & 1 & 1 & & & & \\ 1 & 1 & 1 & 1 & 1 & & & \\ 1 & 1 & 1 & 1 & 1 & 1 & & \\ 1 & 1 & 1 & 1 & 1 & 1 & 1 & 1 \\ 1 & 1 & 1 & 1 & 1 & 1 & 1 & 1 \end{bmatrix}$$

In this model, $N=8$, $K \geq 2$.

6.3.2.9 Model for Command Agents

There are four command agents: Ministry of Health, Health Department in Qinghai, Health Department of GLD, and Health Department in Lanzhou Military Region, and their relationship is as follows (Fig. 6.8, Table 6.8):

The matrix is as follows:

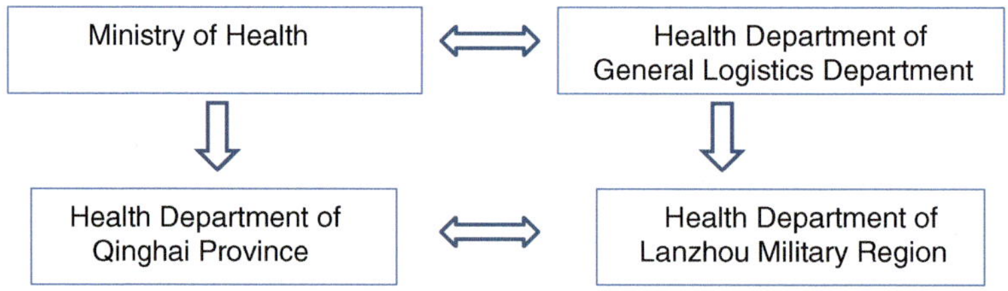

Fig. 6.8 Relationships among command agents

Table 6.8 Relationships among command agents

	Health Department in Qinghai	Health Department in Lanzhou Military Region	Ministry of Health	Health Department of GLD
Health Department in Qinghai	●	●		
Health Department in Lanzhou Military Region	●	●	●	
Ministry of Health		●	●	●
Health Department of GLD			●	●

	n_1	n_2	n_3	n_4
n_1	1	1		
n_2	1	1	1	
n_3		1	1	1
n_4			1	1

In this model, $N=4$, $K=2$.

By the Joint Assembly, the matrix can be converted as follows:

	n_1	n_2	n_3	n_4
n_1	1	1	1	1
n_2	1	1	1	1
n_3	1	1	1	1
n_4	1	1	1	1

In this model, $N=4$, $K=3$.

6.3.2.10 Optimal Model for the Synergy of Rescue Teams

Compared to the two-stage command mode in Wenchuan, the three-level command working mechanism in Yushu was more effective, as it took the four units—Ministry of Health, Health Department of GLD, Health Department of Qinghai Province, and Health Department of Lanzhou Military Region—as a whole, permitting analysis of them as a singular agent. The matrix is as follows:

	n_1	n_2	n_3	n_4	n_5
n_1	1	1	1	1	1
n_2	1	1	1	1	1
n_3	1	1	1	1	1
n_4	1	1	1	1	1
n_5	1	1	1	1	1

In this model, $N=5$, $K=4$.

6.3.2.11 Coordination Matrix in Wenchuan

In Wenchuan, the command system is a three-level command system, so there is more vertical integration and less horizontal coordination.

	n_1	n_2	n_3	n_4	n_5	n_6	n_7	n_8
n_1	1	1						
n_2	1	1	1					
n_3		1	1	1				

n_4			1	1	1			
n_5				1	1	1		
n_6					1	1	1	
n_7						1	1	1
n_8							1	1

In this model, $N=8$, $K=2$.

6.3.2.12 Weak Coordination Matrix

This is a hypothetical situation in which every unit that participated in disaster rescue did not contact each other.

	n_1	n_2	n_3	n_4	n_5	n_6	n_7	n_8
n_1	1	1						
n_2	1	1						
n_3			1	1				
n_4			1	1				
n_5					1	1		
n_6					1	1		
n_7							1	1
n_8							1	1

For example: $N=8$, $K=2$.

6.4 Simulations

6.4.1 Territorial Optimum Performance

Different collaborative models may have effects on fitness landscapes of the system. In order to show the influence, we introduce two indicators to simulate the process, which is the number of territorial optimum values and the territorial optimum performance. The initial performance value of each agent is generated according to random number and varies between 0 and 1. The initial performance value of each agent is evaluated by MATLAB simulation software and can reflect the synergy degree of agents (Rivkin and Siggelkow 2007).

The command coordination mode during the Yushu earthquake medical rescue was the "two-level four-unit" Joint Assembly, and in the Wenchuan earthquake medical rescue, it was a three-level mode, given the different situation (Yu et al. 2011; Zhang et al. 2011). This paper compares and analyzes K values in different types of influence matrices in the table below (Table 6.9).

Under the condition of same degree of interactions, namely, same degree of complexity, different types of interaction modes make the average territorial optimum values of fitness landscape significantly different.

Table 6.9 Territorial optimum values in different influence matrices

K	Strong coordination mode		Weak coordination mode
	Two-level four-unit mode	Three-level command coordination mode	
1	1.8	5.2	5.6
2	3.3	13.8	16.9
3	6.8	27.2	42.5
4	13.5	47.5	78.6

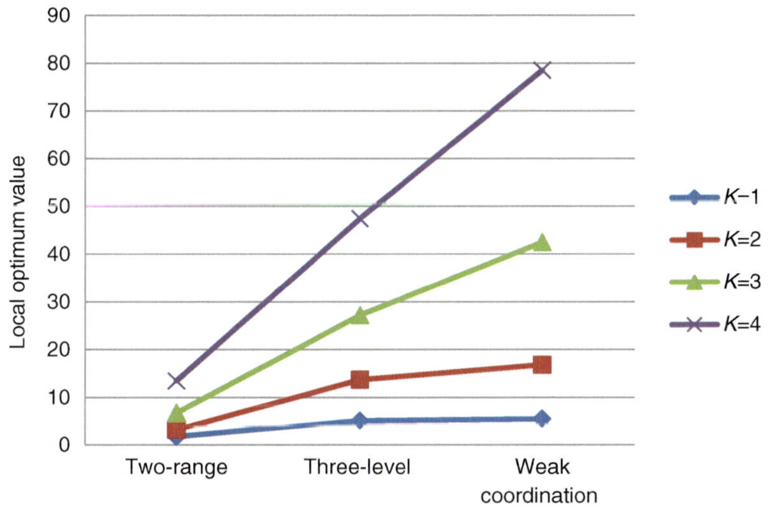

Fig. 6.9 Territorial optimum values in different types of matrices

For example, when $K=2$, the territorial optimum value varies from 3.3 to 16.9, while when $K=4$, it varies from 13.5 to 78.6 (Fig. 6.9).

When the size and the degree of synergistic interaction in the same system, with equivalent conditions of N and K, two levels of command with at least the number of territorial optimum synergy patterns influence the matrix. The collaborative model makes it easier for the system performance to achieve the global optimal level, and the number of weak territorial optimum synergy patterns influences the matrix (Ren and Anumba 2002; Semsar-Kazeroonia and Khorasani 2009; Shehory and Kraus 1998). This kind of collaborative pattern makes it difficult to achieve the optimal level (Fig. 6.10).

6.4.2 *Optimal Average Performance*

With the increase in system complexity, all sorts of influencing matrices of territorial optimal average performance are gradually reduced, the weak coordination model of territorial optimal average performance level is relatively low, and the

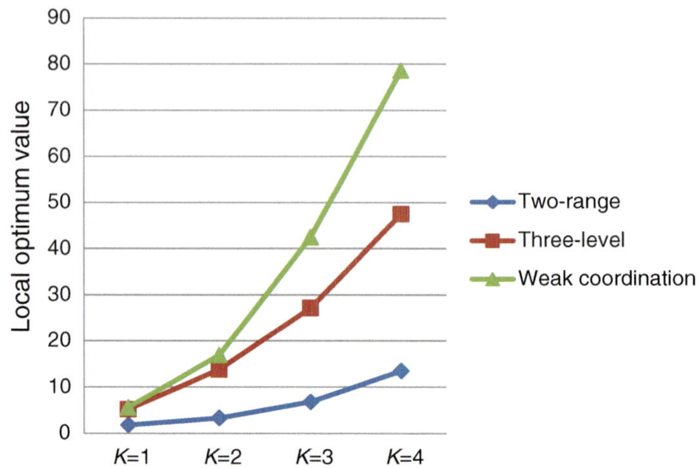

Fig 6.10 Territorial optimum values in different types of matrices

Table 6.10 Optimal average performance in different influencing matrices

K	Strong coordination mode		Weak coordination mode
	Two-level four-unit mode	Three-level mode	
1	0.863	0.858	0.856
2	0.832	0.818	0.813
3	0.812	0.792	0.786
4	0.798	0.772	0.761

two-level four-unit mode influencing matrix has the highest average territorial optimum performance (Table 6.10, Figs. 6.11 and 6.12).

6.5 Summary

Weak coordination

This section summarizes the current situation and problem analysis. The "two-level four-unit" collaborative command mechanism, which was different from the three-level command mechanism in the emergency medical rescue of Wenchuan earthquake, was established in the early stage after the Yushu earthquake. This "two-level four-unit" collaborative command mechanism emphasized the importance of territorial management and emphasized that the commander should be nearer to the rescue teams in the frontline. This mechanism greatly increased the efficiency of resource utilization and decision-making (Akers 1978).

This paragraph summarizes the modeling and simulation. In the matchmaker model, all command agents were divided into three categories, which are P-agent,

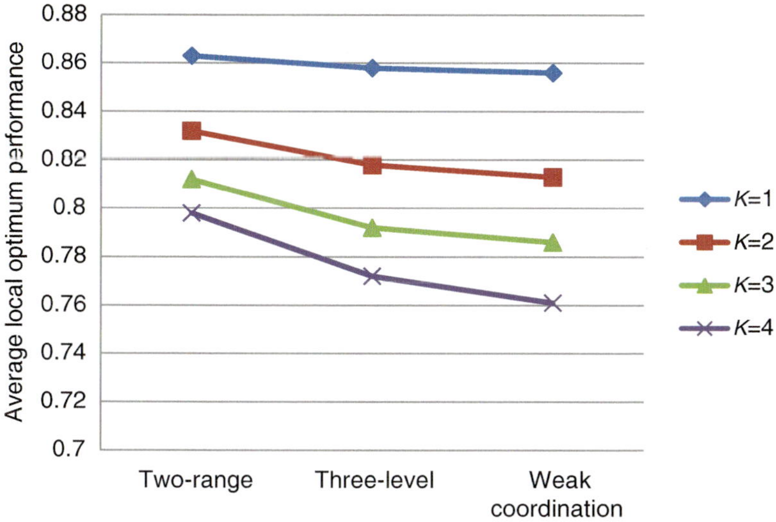

Fig. 6.11 Average territorial optimum performance in different types of matrices

Fig. 6.12 Average territorial optimum performance in different types of matrices

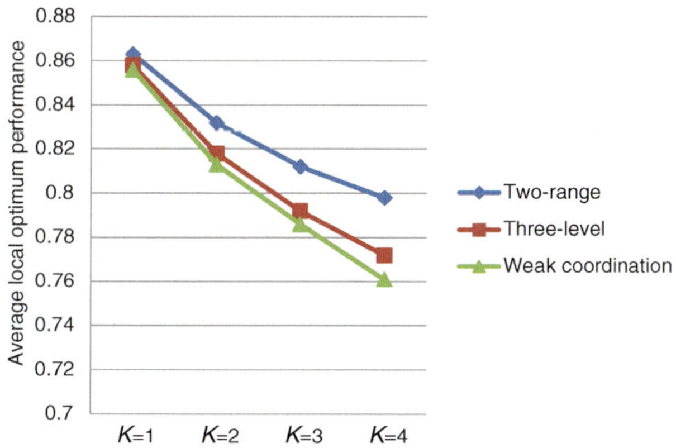

R-agent, and matchmaker. According to the structural characteristics of medical rescue system in Yushu earthquake, the collaborative command could be divided into three types, which were horizontal coordination within the system, vertical coordination within the system, and coordination between the system and the external. All the three types of coordination were strong coordination. There were also three collaborative command models, sequential collaboration, concurrent collaboration, and selective collaboration. Processes of collaborative command in different types of events were shown by combination of these three models in different ways and sequence and could be described by a Petri net mathematical formula (Bryant 1992; Cooper and Hammer 1996). The NK model was competent for describing the complexity of collaborative command system in different types of matrices, and the matrices could be simulated in MATLAB software (Bryant 1992; Clark 2000; Yu and Wang 2010).

When we think of evaluating the influence factors and the effects of collaborative command, there are too many variables related. The variables can be divided into different dimensions and levels. In addition, the agents in collaborative command are people, so the process and effect of collaborative command are normally influenced by people's subjective qualities, and there remain many uncertainties here. In the following work, we should pay more attention to the construction of regulatory framework in order to reduce the possible adverse impact of subjective factors.

References

Abolghasemi H, Poorheidari G, Mehrabi A, et al. Iranian military forces in the Bam earthquake [J]. Mil Med. 2005;170(10):859–61.

Akers SB. Binary decision diagrams. IEEE Trans Comput. 1978;C-27(6):509–16.

Amundson D, Lane D, Ferrara E. Operation aftershock: the U. S. Military Disaster Response to the Yogyakarta Earthquake May through June 2006. Mil Med. 2008;173(3):236–40.

Auerbach PS, Norris RL, Menon AS, et al. Civil–military collaboration in the initial medical response to the earthquake in Haiti [J]. N Engl J Med. 2010;362(10):e32.

Baker MS. Creating order from chaos: part I: triage, initial care, and tactical considerations in mass casualty and disaster response. Mil Med. 2007;172(3):232–6.

Bilham R. Lessons from the Haiti earthquake. Nature. 2010;463:878–9.

Bryant R. Symbolic boolean manipulation with ordered binary decision diagrams. ACM Comput Surveys. 1992;24(3):293–318.

Cavalcante RC, Bittencourt II, et al. A survey of security in multi-agent systems. Exp Syst Appl. 2012;39(5):4835–46.

Chen JQ, Lee SM. An exploratory cognitive DSS for strategic decision making [J]. Decis Supp Syst. 2003;10(36):147–60.

Clark AG. Limits to prediction of phenotypes from knowledge of genotypes. Evol Biol. 2000;32:205–24.

Cooper M, Hammer GL. Synthesis of strategies for crop improvement. In: Cooper M, Hammer GL, editors. Plant adaptation and crop improvement. Wallingford: CAB International; 1996.

Davidson EH, et al. A genomic regulatory network for development. Science. 2002;295:1669–78.

Depew DJ, Weber BH. Darwinism evolving: systems dynamics and the genealogy of natural selection; a Bradford book. Cambridge, MA: The MIT Press; 1996.

Devi S. Helping earthquake-hit Haitithe. Lancet. 2010;375:267–8.

Domres B, Schauwecker HH, Rohrmann K. The German approach to emergency/disaster management. Med Arh. 2000;54(4):201–3.

Hosseini M, Vaz M. The impact of Bam earthquake on substance users in the first 2 weeks: a rapid assessment. J Urban Health Bull New York Acad Med. 2005;82(3):370–7.

Hu G. Robust consensus tracking of a class of second-order multi-agent dynamic systems. Syst Control Lett. 2012;61(1):134–42.

Jennings NR. Controlling cooperative problem solving in industrial multi-agent systems using joint intention [J]. Artif Intell. 1995;75(2):195–240.

Lai WK, Coghill GG. Genetic breeding of control parameters for the Hopfield/Tank neural net[C]// Neural Networks, 1992. IJCNN, Proceedings of International Joint Conference on. IEEE, Baltimore, MD: 1992;4:618–23.

Li S, Wang J, et al. A new framework of consensus protocol design for complex multi-agent systems. Syst Control Lett. 2011;60(1):19–26.

Ligtenberg A, Wachowicz M, et al. A design and application of a multi-agent system for simulation of multi-actor spatial planning. J Environ Manage. 2004;72(1–2):43–55.

Montano BR, Yoon V, et al. Agent learning in the multi-agent contracting system [MACS]. Decis Supp Syst. 2008;45(1):140–9.

Park S, Sugumaran V. Designing multi-agent systems: a framework and application. Exp Syst Appl. 2005;28(2):259–71.

Pastor E, Cortadella J, Roig O. Symbolic analysis of bounded petri nets. IEEE Trans Comput. 2001;50(5):432–48.

Ren Z, Anumba CJ. Learning in multi-agent systems: a case study of construction claims negotiation. Adv Eng Inform. 2002;16(4):265–75.

Rivkin JW, Siggelkow N. Patterned interactions in complex systems: implications for exploration [J]. Management Science. 2007;53(7):1068–85.

Semsar-Kazerooni E, Khorasani K. Multi-agent team cooperation: a game theory approach. Automatica. 2009;45(10):2205–13.

Shehory O, Kraus S. Methods of task allocation via agent coalition formation [J]. Artif Intell. 1998;101(1–2):165–200.

Wagner A. Estimating coarse gene network structure from large-scale gene perturbation data. Genome Res. 2002;21:309–15.

Weinberger ED. Territorial properties of Kauffman's NK model, a tuneably rugged energy landscape. Phys Rev. 1991;44:6399–413. 2002 Wiley Periodicals, Inc. COMPLEXITY 47.

Yager PR. On the inclusion of importance in multi—criteria decision making in the fuzzy set framework [J]. Int J Expert Syst Res Appl. 1992;5:211–28.

Yano M. Genetic and molecular dissection of naturally occurring variation. Curr Opin Plant Biol. 2001;4:130–5.

Yi L, Qi Z, Guofeng S, Xuan L, Lemin L. Simulation of synergetic mechanism in emergency response based on multi-agent method. J Tsing hua Uni v (Sci & Tech), 2010;50(2):165–69.

Yu J, Wang L. Group consensus in multi-agent systems with switching topologies and communication delays. Syst Control Lett. 2010;59(6):340–8.

Yu W, Zheng WX, et al. Second-order consensus in multi-agent dynamical systems with sampled position data. Automatica. 2011;47(7):1496–503.

Zhang L, Liu Y, Liu X, Zhang Y. Rescue efforts management and characteristics of casualties of the Wenchuan Earthquake in China. Emerg Med J. 2011;28(7):618–22.

Zhang J, Cheng L, et al. A multi-agent-based decision support system for bankruptcy contagion effects. Exp Syst Appl. 2012;39(5):5920–34.

Zhu C. Review for renewal lessons and thoughts from Wenchuan earthquake medical rescue. J Evidence Based Med. 2009;2(3):150–1.

Chapter 7
Modeling Location and Distribution of Medical Support Institutions

Yang Ge, Yuan Liu, Yipeng Lv, and Lulu Zhang

Abstract This chapter contains four parts. In order to understand the modeling of the location and distribution of medical rescue institutions, this chapter presents an introduction to the location and distribution optimization of medical supporting institutions, the data resource used in location and distribution optimization of medical support institutions model, construction of the location and distribution optimization of medical support institutions model, and analysis of the location and distribution optimization of medical support institutions model. The first section presents the background, objective, and significance as well as the technical route and design. The second section describes the utilization of the current data resource and data source from field surveys. The third section illustrates the parameters of the location and distribution optimized model of medical support institutions and construction of the location and distribution optimized model of medical support institutions. The last section provides a systemic simulation and describes the utilization of the location and distribution optimization of medical support institutions model. The summary discusses the optimized location and distribution plan of medical rescue institutions, distribution optimization of medical institutions in regional forces, and distribution optimization of medicine supply institutions in regional joint service forces.

Y. Ge • Y. Liu • Y. Lv
Department of Military Health Service, College of Military Health Service, Second Military Medical University, Yangpu, Shanghai, China

L. Zhang, PhD (✉)
Department of Military Health Service, College of Military Health Service, Second Military Medical University, Shanghai, China
e-mail: zllrmit@aliyun.com

© Springer Science+Business Media Dordrecht 2016
L. Zhang (ed.), *Modeling the Injury Flow and Treatment after Major Earthquakes*, DOI 10.1007/978-94-017-7527-4_7

7.1 Introduction to Location and Distribution Optimization of Medical Support Institutions

7.1.1 *Background*

7.1.1.1 Location Optimization of Medical Support Institutions

Relevant Concepts

The location of medical support institutions refers to the address chosen for medical support institutions. Actually, however, analysis of the location of medical support institutions focuses on the expansion of institutions and dispose districts. The aim of optimizing the location of medical support institutions is to choose the corresponding dispose districts through distinguishing among the functions and tasks of various medical supporting institutions, thus facilitating the completion of the task and, ultimately, achieving the goal of medical rescue.

The medical support institutions have their respective mandates and so the significance of choosing locations varies. The location optimization of medical supporting institutions starts from the location decision unit, which is associated with the "wartime deployment" problem of medical service command and securing the decision problem matrix (Baker 2007). It focuses on the study of location optimization issues under uncertainty through screening of the location of medical support institutions under emergency and wartime conditions in order to select representative medical support institutions as model targets and conduct related studies on optimization modeling.

Location Optimization of Medical Supporting Institutions Under Emergencies

Currently, from SARS to the avian flu, there are a growing number of public health emergencies, which have necessitated new work requirements for public health preparedness. As a medical support institution, the institution should not only be responsible for medical rescue tasks but also bear the social and national protection missions of public health emergencies. Accordingly, this paper presents the issues related to medical rescue under emergency conditions. As a place for medical support institutions to organize the implementation of security, the dispose districts of medical support institutions and their expansion play an important role in the entire emergency medical rescue and protection. While analyzing the characteristics of medical rescue tasks under emergency conditions, occurrence regularities and treatment requirements of public health emergencies should be considered aiming at the security tasks of various medical supporting institutions, and the optimization issues of medical rescue protection agencies should be screened.

Medical institutions under emergency conditions are the emergency mobile medical institutions composed by the mobile medical services in the military hospitals, i.e., the prebuilt medical resources by the military (Abolghasemi et al. 2005; Amundson et al. 2008). Under emergency conditions, the institutions deal with public health emergencies, including providing accommodation for the wounded, classification processing, and medical care tasks. Location optimization of medical institutions is, under emergency conditions, intended to select the appropriate region to configure and launch medical institutions, in order to facilitate the smooth progress of medical treatment tasks, guarantee a higher quality of medical treatment, and improve the cure rate and reduce mortality of the sick and wounded.

Relevant Concepts of the Optimal Distribution of Medical Support Institutions

The distribution of medical support institutions refers to the configuration of resources within a certain area, and here, it refers to the layout of medical support institutions within a given area (war zones, divisions, provincial military, etc.). Optimal distribution refers to the problem of appropriately laying out resources in a certain area. It uses the optimal method to establish an optimal model in order to allow the distribution of resources to be in an optimal state within a region. The goal is to spatially determine the optimal allocation and utilization of resources.

The distribution of medical support institutions belongs to the realm of the distribution of health protection entities. According to the different functions of medical support institutions, the distribution issues are screened to three categories, i.e., medical evacuation, health and epidemic prevention, and medicinal herb protection (Kang et al. 2012; Lulu et al. 2012). As there are many medical evacuation institutions, the distribution issues are distributed into military hospitals (i.e., base hospitals and rear hospitals) and grassroots medical institutions (i.e., division medical aid stations, brigade medical aid stations, regiment medical aid stations, and battalion and company rescue units). This chapter introduces the distribution optimization issues using military hospitals and medical supply agencies as an example.

7.1.2 Objective and Significance

This project is the subtopic of *Research on Methods and Standards of Military Health Resource Allocation* (01z101-1), one of the Army "Fifteenth" Medical Research Key Planning Projects. According to the theory of military health resource allocation, spatial decision support system (SDSS), and computer software development technology, using preliminary studies of the task force as references, this thesis builds the optimized distribution model of regional medical resources, reveals the optimized distribution configuration mechanism of regional army medical resources, proposes the optimized distribution configuration plan of regional army medical resources, and finalizes the reasonable distribution and utilization efficiency of army medical resources. All of these findings are based on the medical service demand and utilization of military personnel, the status and prediction of regional military medical resource allocation, and the situation analysis of regional military medical resource distribution. The research and development of the software "Weijun No. 1" was conducted with the system of regional military medical resource allocation decisions—specifically, the distribution of the support system (RMMRODA-DSS), docks with the optimized microscopic military medical resource decision support systems developed by the task force during the same period as "Weijun No. 1," the hospital information system "Junwei No. 1," which was uniformly developed and implemented by the entire army, and "Red Star No. 1," which was developed and implemented by cooperating organizations, thereby realizing the information management of regional military medical resources. Therefore, the theoretical system of military health resource allocation can be improved in order to provide a basis and decision-making tools for the reorganization of regional military health resources.

7.1.3 Technical Route and Design

For various categories of medical support institutions, the launch of institutions and location issues are related to a variety of factors (Ofer et al. 2010; Zhang et al. 2010). One of the important factors is the impact of the location of medical support institutions. This chapter is based on using a model that is relatively practical and easy to implement to solve various location issues of institutions.

Through analyzing the impact of medical support institution locations, and using analytic hierarchy process (AHP) to determine the weight value of each factor, based on a geographic information system (GIS) database, the combat zone can then be divided into several smaller areas. Based on the weight values of each influencing factor carried out by AHP and using the GIS spatial analysis functions, these qualitative and quantitative factors and other relevant information in the smallest unit of an internal location in the approximate geographical location can then be determined. Then, a plurality of candidate points of the weight value information will be obtained, and through the minimum weight limit identified by the decision maker, the corresponding candidate points can be obtained. Then, according to the minimum distance from the medical support institution to each object to protect, the best alternative solution can be found.

In different external environments, both under emergency and wartime conditions, the location influencing factors and security objects may change accordingly. Therefore, as long as the changes in location factors under different conditions have been discovered, quantitative and/or qualitative analyses are conducted with regard to various influencing factors, and both quantitative and qualitative factors are combined using the given model, a better location plan can be obtained.

7.2 Data Resource Used in the Location and Distribution Optimization of Medical Support Institutions Model

7.2.1 Utilization of the Current Data Resource

The thesis uses field investigation data of the "Research on Criteria and Methodology of Military Health Resource Allocation" task force for herb security agencies in a given war zone (medicine warehouses, medical supply stations, and instrument control institute for drug and instrument control) as well as security object units (medical institutions above the regimental). It includes the distribution of supply agencies, human resources, and supplies, in addition to the distribution of security object units and security relationships.

7.2.1.1 Collection of the Current Data Resource

The current data included local demographic data and socioeconomic development indicators; computer network statistics from health information management systems within the region; various types of conventional statistical report data of the health statistics departments; all types of health statistics yearbooks and bulletins (1998–2002); conventional statistical report data of various heath sectors; China Health Statistics Yearbook (1998–2002); all kinds of methodology monographs, application models, and software; and health policies, guidelines, conference materials, different kinds of books, and literature related to allocation of resources at the national level (military).

7.2.1.2 Information Management System of Military Medical Institutions

Using the computer network of *Information Management System of Military Medical Institutions*, this thesis conducted a survey of military hospitals in a war zone and has gathered basic data from 23 military hospitals, central hospitals, and general hospitals, including institutions, human resources, bedding configuration, and utilization conditions.

7.2.2 Data Source from Field Surveys

7.2.2.1 Field Investigation Data

All the data are from the field investigation of the project, including all 23 second- and third-level general hospitals in a certain war zone. This thesis collected the five categories of exogenous medical resources from various hospitals from 1998 to

2002. It focused on military medical institutions, manpower, bed space, equipment, funding elements of resources, and emergency medical service and the situation of maneuvering forces.

7.2.2.2 Expert Consultation Survey

This thesis conducted surveys on the heads of military hospitals and managers of health administrative authorities in a certain war zone and has learned the basic situation of hospitals and emergency mobile medical services. Scores of matching degrees were assigned to unexpected events and emergency mobile medical services, and the weight coefficients were determined. Among them, there are 18 agency administrative staff (23.08 %), 23 hospital directors (29.49 %), and 37 health professional workers (47.44 %).

7.2.2.3 Collection of Documents

Paper documents included relevant policy documents from herb joint logistics support. Relevant documents issued under the General Logistics Department of Health include *Basic Health Equipment Standard Under the Army Division*, *Basic Standards of Army Herb for Readiness Under the Army Division*, *Opinions on Strengthening Military Medical Supply Management*, and the files *Jinan War Zone Medical Supply Relationship and Supply Channels* provided by the Bureau of Herbs, which is affiliated with the General Logistics Department of Health. *Logistics academic* and *PLA Medical Service magazine*, along with related literature, were also analyzed.

For electronic literature, journals searched included "PLA Hospital Management Journal," "Military Medical Journal of South China," "Pharmaceutical Care and Practice," "System Engineering Theory and Practice," and "Management Engineering Journal." Nearly 200 relevant articles were obtained, and then inductive and summary analyses were conducted.

7.2.2.4 Relevant Literature and Data Use

To study the allocation of medical resources in the regional military, existing documents and information are also important. These include the following:

- Healthcare reform plans and reports of the General Logistics Department
- Construction status and analysis reports of military hospitals in a certain war zone, speeches of the heads, and related materials, monographs, and literature
- Preliminary research data of the task force and findings regarding macroscopic allocation of health resources
- SDSS and relevant information of software development technology

7.3 Construction of the Location and Distribution Optimization of Medical Support Institutions Model

7.3.1 Parameters of the Location and Distribution Optimized Model of Medical Support Institutions

7.3.1.1 Parameter Establishment of the Location Optimization of Medical Support Institutions Model

The parameters involved in the location optimization of medical support institutions model include the weight value of influencing factors, weight value lower limit of the candidate point, quantized values of influencing factors, and the distance between institutions and security institutions.

Weight Value of Influencing Factors

Influencing factors can be obtained by expert consultation and other means, and then according to pairwise comparison matrices of various influencing factors, through building hierarchical analysis model and using AHP, the weight values of different location choices of each influencing factor can be obtained.

Weight Value Lower Limit of the Candidate Point

This refers to process by which the candidate point with the smaller weight value is excluded from the optimal solution after obtaining each candidate point. This is done in order to narrow the scope of location choice, given the weight value lower limit of candidate point. Through this method, the selection can be narrowed, and operations can be reduced. In accordance with all the candidate point circumstances, the policymakers generally construct a weight value lower limit.

Quantized Values of Influencing Factors

The decision-makers determine these values depending on the specific requirements of various security institutions and specific combating circumstances.

Security Distance

This is obtained from measuring the distance of the drawing by GIS. It can be divided into the shortest path and straight-line distance on a drawing and is mainly based for functions of the GIS platform.

7.3.1.2 Influencing Factors of Medical Support Institution Locations

Regarding the model of ideas regarding the location optimization of medical support institutions, it has been mentioned that AHP can be used to analyze factors that influence the location of medical support institutions and to set up an analytic hierarchy model of medical supporting institutions. Therefore, the analysis must be conducted on the influencing factors of the screened medical support institutions under emergency and wartime conditions in order to determine the optimal location using GIS technology.

Medical rescue institutions are the principal institutions for contingency and wartime treatment of the sick and wounded under emergency and wartime conditions. External environment, treatment institutions themselves, and treatment targets affect their locations. The specific influencing factors include the main operational direction, combat attrition rate, emergency geographical disease composition, and evacuation roads.

For the geographical configuration choice of medical support institutions, an optimal model of location will permit discussion on the location optimization problems of medical supporting institutions through the established location theoretical model using GIS. It will also provide a rapid decision method for medical support under uncertainty. Thus, it can reveal the location optimization mechanism of medical support institutions and provide decision support for location optimization of medical support institutions under uncertainty.

7.3.1.3 Parameter Establishment of Location Optimization Models of Medical Supporting Institutions

Two main parameters must be set up, namely, the load of medical support institutions and the effective serving radius (ESR). ESR is used to optimize the distance between medical support institutions and the concerned troops, and demand of the concerned troops and load of medical support institutions are used to optimize the scope of medical support institutions. The parameters can be set according to the different levels of medical support institutions.

Effective Service Radius

ESR refers to the geographical coverage of securing people in mass when the health resources are at maximum efficiency within the medical support institutions. ESR is the best match point between health supply capacity and people's health service demand. The greater its coverage, the greater the service capability of the medical supporting institution and the greater its radius. Conversely, the smaller its coverage, the lesser the service capability of the medical supporting institution and the smaller its radius.

The fundamental factors that determine ESR of medical support institutions are the support capabilities of medical support institutions and population health demand characteristics. If the geographical scope and service network covered by medical support institutions are excessive, its service capabilities will be in short supply. If its own scale is not expanded or its capacity to offer health services is not enhanced, the quality and level of health services will be reduced, and it cannot meet people's health service demands. On the other hand, if the geographical scope covered is too small and there is surplus service capability, then it will detrimentally affect the efficiency of health resources. Thus, the best ESR should be sought after in order to achieve a state of not wasting resources while still meeting the health service demands of the people, thereby maximizing the utilization efficiency of health resources.

ESR of Military Hospitals

The main task of military hospitals is to treat evacuated patients from higher-level hospitals. According to "Medical Institution Regulations" and "Medical Institutions Guiding Principles" by the State Council, the ESR can be determined for demand features regarding demand for medical services at different levels in the army. For the distribution relationship across all levels of the military hospitals in a certain war zone, after access to information and consulting experts, this thesis sets the ESR of garrison hospitals as 50 km and the ESR of central hospitals as 100 km.

ESR of Herb Security Institutions

After the army has implemented joint logistics, the joint logistics herb security institutions include two agencies, namely, the medicinal warehouse and medical supply station. The functions of the two institutions are different. However, some of the war zones have combined depot and filling duties, and their functions may overlap. Currently, a war zone generally establishes 1–2 professional medicinal warehouses, and every medicinal warehouse has medical supply stations. The effective protection radius of medical supply institutions refers to the maximum distance it can protect within its capabilities. The radius is determined by its ability to protect itself, geographical features, demand of the security object, and other factors. If the geographical scope and service network covered by medical supply institutions are excessive, its security capabilities will be in short supply, thus leading to the sacrifice of quality and effectiveness in order to complete security tasks. Ultimately, such institutions will not be able to meet the mass demands of the army. On the other hand, if the geographical scope covered by medical supply institutions is too small and there is surplus security capability, then it will seriously affect the utilization efficiency of herb institution resources. It can be seen that the effective protection radius of medical supply institutions should be determined in order to achieve the state of not wasting resources while still meeting the herb demands of the army. This will maximize the utilization efficiency of medical supply institutions.

According to the current circumstances of joint logistics medical supply institutions in the war zone, the medicinal warehouse can be divided into two categories, namely, professional warehouse and branch warehouse within the comprehensive warehouse. Professional medicinal warehouses currently undertake the heaviest supporting tasks in the war zone. The sole professional medicinal warehouse supports the herb security of joint logistics services and arms. From the perspective of supporting capabilities, it has the maximum effective protection radius.

With reference to the distribution relationship among all medical supply institutions in the war zone, after referring to information and consulting experts, this thesis sets the effective protection radius of professional medicinal warehouses as 200 km and the effective protection radius of medical supply stations as 150 km.

Load of Protection

Load intent refers to the external resistance that machinery or driving machine must overcome. It is then extended to the requirements mentioned for the operational capacity of a system. In this thesis, it refers to the support capabilities of medical support institutions within the region (i.e., the maximum number of people that the institutions can protect under certain conditions with health service needs). This thesis takes a certain war zone as an example in order to explain.

Protection Load of Military Hospitals

The load of military hospitals refers to the hospital's ability to treat patients per unit time, that is, the ability to protect soldiers of military hospitals. It is mainly determined by the bedding scales of military hospitals. Military hospitals do not only protect the army—they also are tasked with serving ordinary people. According to the bedding staff principle of military hospitals, the hospital chooses prepared beds as the load index of military hospitals.

A certain war zone has a total population of 504,319 people and 4310 sheets of bedding, with an average security of 117 people per bed. Considering the utilization efficiency of bedding resources in military hospitals in the war zone and demand conditions of military medical services, combined with the functions and tasks of military hospitals in this war zone, via access to information and consultation with experts, the security capability per bed is selected to be 150 people in central hospitals and 120 people in garrison hospitals. The security capability of various levels of military hospitals in the war zone is then calculated accordingly.

Load of Protection of Herb Security Institutions

Medical supply institutions, according to their own scales and various protection tasks, protect the herbs for security object units. When discussing the effective protection radius of herb security institutions, the protection capability of medical supply institutions has been mentioned, and the institutions must launch herb protection work according to their own protection capability. They should do so "within their capabilities," that is, conduct the protection work within their protection capacity (i.e., load of protection).

For medical supply agencies, their protection capacity is affected by various factors, including annual medicine turnover volume, storage capacity, staffing, handling capacity, transport capacity, annual turnover amount, and so forth. Therefore, at the current level of the war zone, when the medical supply management organ (Medicine Office of the Ministry of Health, Joint Logistics Department) is assessing the security functions of joint logistics medical supply agencies, it makes calculations given the annual total medicine protection volume of medical supply agencies. Therefore, after calculating the annual total medicine protection volume of medical supply agencies, the load of protection of herb security institutions is obtained.

Security Demands

Demand mainly refers to the volume of demand that the security object requests of medical support institutions. Demand for medical services can generally be determined using biweekly prevalence rate, that is, the number of people in system forces multiplied by the biweekly prevalence rate of force personnel in the army. Herb demand is relatively complex and there is a wide variety. However, there is a need to find a single, representative, and unified parameter that can measure the demand to represent the volume of demand. The army has corresponding annual health expenditures, and all herb purchases use this expenditure. Therefore, according to the analysis above, we utilized the amount of money to measure the size of the herb demand in the army. Focusing on a certain troop, find the product volume application of herbs in recent years, convert it into the corresponding price in accordance with the amount, and use the arithmetic average as the amount of money the average annual army herb demand. This method has greater requirements of historical data and has the feature of predictability. According to this idea, and with further consideration, we can set up a standard parameter "annual demand for herbs per capita." When calculating army demand, it is simply multiplied by the total number of security. For differences in manning quotas and types for various troops, attributions for "annual demand for herbs per capita" can be classified differently for different types of troops. It is then easy to determine the medicinal demand of the forces.

7.3.2 Construction of the Location and Distribution Optimized Model of Medical Support Institutions

7.3.2.1 Structure of Analytic Hierarchy

Given the various influencing factors of medical supporting institution locations, this chapter does not list influencing factors of various types of institutions but, rather, uses only a field medicine warehouse as an example to discuss.

Table 7.1 Field medicine warehouse location factors pairwise comparison matrices

	Near the main attack road	Near the command post	Near the railroad terminal	Near major highways
Near the main attack road	1	3	2	1
Near the command post	0.3	1	0.5	0.3
Near the railroad terminal	0.5	2	1	0.5
Near major highways	1	3	2	1

The influencing factors of field medicine warehouse locations is very complex, including geographical factors, environmental factors, factors of medical supply itself, and so on. The following should be noted when setting up and expanding: (1) good transportation conditions but avoiding military targets that could possibly be attacked by the enemy, (2) better set in front of nearby important bridges and main roads, (3) take full advantage of protective equipment on the spot, and (4) easy to camouflage, conceal, and distribute alerts. Based on the duties of field operation medicinal warehouses, after access to information and consulting experts, this thesis selects factors influencing the choosing of field medicine warehouse locations and builds the analytic hierarchy structure model. The goal layer refers to locations of field operation medicinal warehouses. The criterion layer includes two factors, namely, benefit to medical supply and benefit to medicine safety. Each of these factors is divided into three sub-criteria. The former includes near the main attack road, near the railroad terminal, near the command post, and near major highways, whereas the latter includes easy to be hidden, away from rivers, and avoiding major military targets and low-lying lands (Table 7.1).

7.3.2.2 Factors Affecting the Weight

Factors Affecting the Hierarchical Analysis Matrix

Constructing the judgment matrix of each layer can help to determine the weight coefficient (from the top to lower) of the same layer. Here, we assume that the factors on the current layer are $A_1 \cdots A_n$, and the relevant upper layer factor is C. In this case, factors from $A_1 \cdots A_n$ can be compared in pairs, thus obtaining the number a_{ij}. If $A=\left(a_{ij}\right)_{n\times n}$, then A is the corresponding factor of $A_1 \cdots A_n$ to the judgment matrix of upper layer factor C. If the greatest characteristic root for A is written as $\lambda_{\max}$, then its corresponding eigenvectors $w=\left(w_i, \&, w_n\right)T$. $(w_i, \ldots, w_n)$ gives the factors $A_1 \cdots A_n$ an order of significance based on factor C. Accordingly, we can draw the layer relative to the upper layer weight coefficient. The maximum of judgment matrix eigenvalues and the factor weight calculation formula is obtained by using the root method (7.1, 7.2)

$$A=\begin{matrix} & \begin{matrix} A_1 & \cdots & A_n \end{matrix} \\ \begin{matrix} A_1 \\ \vdots \\ A_n \end{matrix} & \begin{pmatrix} a_{11} & \cdots & a_{1n} \\ \vdots & & \vdots \\ a_{n1} & \cdots & a_{nn} \end{pmatrix} \end{matrix} \Rightarrow w_i=\frac{\overline{w}_i}{\sum_{i=1}^{n}\overline{w}_i} \Rightarrow \overline{w}_i \approx \sqrt[n]{\prod_{j=1}^{n} a_{ij}} \tag{7.1}$$

$$\lambda_{\max} \approx \frac{1}{n}\sum_{i=1}^{n}\frac{(Aw)_i}{w_i} \tag{7.2}$$

After calculating the maximum characteristic root, we then calculate the same layer of all factors to the highest level (total goal) in order of significance. This process is conducted in order from the highest level to the lowest level; accordingly, we can obtain the weight value of all six sub-criteria contributing to the goal layer after standardized process. Finally, we use the formula to calculate both CI and CR for a consistency check.

If the results comply with the consistency check, the weight value of standardized sub-criteria can be obtained relative to the goal level (six factors the total weight value of six factors amounts to 1). The weight coefficient will be applied to the spatial data analysis function of GIS.

Factors Affecting the Attainment of Weight Values

Based on the spatial data analysis and display function of GIS, the location of the targeted area can be roughly divided into several communities, and the geographical center of each community is used as the coordinates for the community. By using the spatial information analysis function of GIS, the relevant information can be obtained via the geographic center of the analytic hierarchy structure model concerning its various factors. Upon obtaining the result of the weight coefficients of the factors relative to the goal layer, we can obtain the weight value of all factors relative to sub-criteria about each of the geographic centers via the spatial data analysis function of GIS. Then, the weight of each factor can be amounted to the total of all factors (maximum 1, minimum 0).

Some of the quantitative factors of the sub-criteria must be quantized before the spatial data analysis function can be conducted with GIS. Distances must be specified with regard to how far it is from the main direction of the road, main roads, railways, docks, command post, rivers, and major military target distance. These factors must then be quantized before using GIS to analyze. Qualitative factors, such as ability to be hidden, can be directly obtained according to the attribute of each point in the GIS database. In short, the goal is to make the spatial analysis function of GIS identify the degree of consistency of various factors in the sub-criterion layer.

When various sub-criteria factors have been quantized, the corresponding information of each geographic center can be obtained via the spatial analysis function of GIS. Afterward, the corresponding quantized degree of conformity for each factor will lead to the weight value for each geographic center. The specific rules are as follows: if it is close to some factor, such as a road near a main attack direction, with a quantitative range of 2–5 km, then its weight value with a quantitative range of 2–5 km will be equal to the result from the analytic hierarchy process to calculate the factor weights; otherwise, it will be 0. If it is away from some factor, such as a road away from the military target, with a quantitative range of 3–5 km, then its weight value with a quantitative range of 3–5 km will be equal to the result from the analytic hierarchy process to calculate the factor weights; otherwise, it will be 0.

7.3.2.3 Establishment of the Optimal Plan

Establishment of the Objective Function

Based on analyzing the importance of each factor and with "rapid" security as the goal, the best location is screened by objective function (i.e., the fastest security speed). After obtaining the synthetic weight of each point within the region, this thesis will choose a number of *m* points as the candidate points for choosing the location with the rule that the synthetic weight is greater than a specified value (based on the specific circumstances set by decision-makers). Then, the objective function of the sum of the shortest distance between security institutions and a number of *n* demand institutions is as follows (7.3):

$$\text{Min } U = \sum_{j=1}^{n} \sqrt{\left(x_i - x_j\right)^2 + \left(y_i - y_j\right)^2} \tag{7.3}$$

Among them, the coordinates of the *i*th security institution candidate point are (x_i, y_i) (the coordinate value is obtained by using GIS geographic center of gravity); the coordinates of the *j*th demand institution are (x_j, y_j) (the coordinates are known in advance, as the locations of these institutions have identified their specific locations prior to siting).

Solving the Objective Function

According to the objective function, we can solve the distance sum of the shortest path between each candidate point and *n* known demand institutions. Then, *m* distance sums of the shortest path can be obtained, and we take the candidate point with the minimum value to be the solution of the model, which is the optimal plan for location.

The Shortest Path Method

This model uses the simple straight-line distance on a drawing to calculate the distance sum. Using GIS spatial analysis function and graph theory method to obtain the shortest path between two institutions has been applied in contemporary practice. The more commonly used method is that of Dijkstra.

7.3.2.4 The Modeling Steps of the Location Optimization Model of Medical Support Institutions

The model is divided into two parts. The first is the establishment of the security relationship matrix. Based on the ESR of medical supporting institutions at various levels, we determine the distribution relationship between medical support institutions and security objects within the region. The second is the establishment of the distribution optimization model, that is, the optimization of the distribution relationship between medical support institutions and security objects within the region.

Establishment of Relationship Matrix

According to location distribution conditions of medical support institutions and security objects within the region, the ESR of medical support institutions at each level can be determined. Then, the relationship matrix of the distance between medical support institutions and security objects can be established and determine the distribution relationship between them (i.e., whether the security object is within the ESR of the medical support institution).

Assuming there are m security objects, which are represented by b_1, b_2, … $b_{m,}$ n military medical supporting institutions, which are represented by y_1, y_2, … y_n, we can calculate the following:

The distances from the first security object b_1 to all the medical supporting institutions are d_{11}, d_{12}, d_{13}, … d_{1n}.

The distances from the second security object b_2 to all the medical supporting institutions are d_{21}, d_{22}, d_{23}, … d_{2n}.

………………………………

The distances from the mth security object b_1 to all the medical supporting institutions are d_{m1}, d_{m2}, $d_{m3,}$ … d_{mn}.

Assuming the ESRs of all the medical support institutions within the region are r_1, r_2, … r_n, we can establish the following two matrices and subsequently perform the subtraction:

$$\begin{pmatrix} r_1, r_2, \ldots\ldots r_n \\ r_1, r_2, \ldots\ldots r_n \\ \ldots\ldots\ldots\ldots\ldots \\ r_1, r_2, \ldots\ldots r_n \end{pmatrix} \begin{pmatrix} d_{11}, d_{12}, d_{13} \ldots\ldots d_{1n} \\ d_{21}, d_{22}, d_{33} \ldots\ldots d_{2n} \\ \ldots\ldots\ldots\ldots\ldots\ldots\ldots\ldots \\ d_{m1}, d_{m2}, d_{m3} \ldots\ldots d_{mn} \end{pmatrix}$$

$$A = \begin{pmatrix} a_{11}, & a_{12}, & a_{13}, & \ldots\ldots a_{1n} \\ a_{21}, & a_{22}, & a_{23}, & \ldots\ldots a_{2n} \\ \ldots\ldots & \ldots\ldots & \ldots\ldots & \\ a_{m1}, & a_{m2}, & a_{m3}, & \ldots\ldots a_{mn} \end{pmatrix}$$

It is easy to see that in matrix A, the element a_{ij} refers to the ESR of the jth health institution and the distance between the ith systematic security object and the jth health institution.

If $a_{ij} \geq 0$, it means that the ith security object is within the ESR of the jth health institution.

If $a_{ij} < 0$, it means that the ith security object is not within the ESR of the jth health institution.

In this case, the positive and negative elements in each row case clearly show whether the security object is within the ESR of the health institution.

Building the Optimal Model

1. If the security object is distributed in the ESR of a sole medical support institution, then the security object belongs to this medical support institution. Identify all the security objects in the relationship matrix and determine its attribution.
2. If the security object is distributed in the ESR of two medical support institutions, it indicates that the security object will choose one of the two to be the medical support institution. All such forces must be identified in the relationship matrix. Then, we indicate the security object within the ESR of the two medical support institutions to be security object sequence A (without regard to order), determine the security object in the ESR of the same two medical support institutions, and solve the problem according to the following model. After solving the solution—that is, after obtaining the attribution of the security object— it can be removed from sequence A. Repeat the steps above until sequence A is empty, that is, complete all distributions in the ESR of two medical support institutions.
3. If the security object is distributed in the ESR of three or more than three medical support institutions, it indicates that the security object will choose one to be the medical support institution among three or more medical support institutions. The approach is similar to the ESR of two medical support institutions and will be solved by the following model:

$$\text{Objective function} : (i = 1, 2, 3 \ldots\ldots s,\ j = 1, 2, 3 \ldots\ldots t) \tag{7.4}$$

$$\text{Min } Z = \sum_{j=1}^{t} \sum_{j=1}^{s} X_{ij} d_{ij}$$

d_{ij} refers to the distance from the ith security object to the jth medical support institution.

s refers to the number of security objects in the cross.
t refers to the number of medical support institutions in the cross.
Constraint condition:
Due to the special nature of the army population distribution and protection capacities of various levels of medical support institutions, and to make the size of the medical support institutions consistent with the protection load and achieve rational distribution of resources, the protection load is set to be the constraint condition of the model:

$$\begin{cases} x_{11}n_1 + x_{21}n_2 \ldots\ldots + x_{s1}n_s \ £\ F_1 \\ x_{12}n_1 + x_{22}n_2 \ldots\ldots + x_{s1}n_s \ £\ F_2 \\ \ldots\ldots\ldots\ldots\ldots\ldots\ldots\ldots\ldots\ldots \\ x_{1t}n_1 + x_{2t}n_2 \ldots\ldots + x_{st}n_s \ £\ F_t \end{cases}$$

$$(i=1,2\ldots\ldots\ldots\ldots s; j=1,2\ldots\ldots\ldots\ldots t) \tag{7.5}$$

$$\sum_{j=1}^{t} X_{ij} = 1$$

$$X_{ij} = 0\begin{cases} 1\ldots\text{No. } i \text{ security object is affiliated with No.} j \\ \text{militarymedical support institution} \\ \text{No. } i \text{ security object is not affiliated with No.} j \\ \text{militarymedical supporting institution} \end{cases}$$

n_j represents the demand for health services of j security object.
F_i represents the load of j medical support institution.

4. If the security object is distributed in the ESR of various medical support institutions, and each medical support institution exceeds the security load, the model has no solution; if the security object is not distributed in any of the ESRs of various medical support institutions, the model has no solution. At this time, not considering the load of medical support institutions, the security object belongs to the nearest medical support institution.

7.4 Analysis of the Location and Distribution Optimization of Medical Support Institutions Model

7.4.1 Systemic Simulation

7.4.1.1 The Model and Systemic Analysis of Medical Support Institution's Location and Distribution

The location and distribution optimization of medical support institutions model, which mainly targets the uncertain location and distribution under conditions of uncertainty and wartime, is a theoretical combination of qualitative and quantitative factors. The model analyzes the factors affecting the location and distribution of medical support institutions by using GIS to access weight values of various factors based on the quantification of those factors. The use of GIS can allocate comprehensive weight values for each geographic center according to different situations and decision-makers' preference to choose a minimum comprehensive weight value with higher weight values then becoming the alternative location. Through the establishment of the objective function of the shortest distance between medical support institution and security agencies and the shortest distance of the objective function, the center point of the objective function can be achieved from alternatives, thus ultimately reaching the optimal configuration plan of different medical support institutions.

7.4.1.2 Location Optimization Mechanism

The mechanism is the interpretation of the model, and it is also the exploratory recognition based on the theoretical assumptions of a given issue. The location optimization mechanism of emergency and wartime medical support institutions is based on the location optimization mechanism. Through the construction of the model, we can obtain the location optimization mechanism of medical support institution in order to attain the goal of quick and effective security under emergency and wartime conditions. According to various factors contributing to the location configuration of medical support institutions under different conditions (emergency and wartime) along with the distinction in security objects, the optimized location plan for medical support institutions can be achieved by the hypothesis of ignoring the cost and security objects of medical support institutions, the guidelines of quick security and comprehensive thoughts, the constraint of the minimal weight value of factors in choosing alternative locations, and the principle of shortest distance between medical support institutions and security objects.

The mechanism is the interpretation of the model in that the location and distribution optimization of medical support institutions model via the construction of the model is to obtain the optimized distribution and use of medical support institutions, as well as to determine the optimal protection relationship between medical support institutions and security objects. Optimizing decisions based on two major systems given the hypothesis of not changing the geographic location of medical support services requires the spatial dimension used to optimize the decision-making process. One of these systems is the medical support institutions (location radius, effective service, and support capability), and the other is the security object (location and demand for health services). Following the principle of "zoning protection, toward optimal convenience" and the constraint condition of the medical support institutions' security load, the spatial distribution of medical support institutions can realize its optimal status within its appropriate workload and the shortest distance range.

7.4.2 *Utilization of the Location and Distribution Optimization of Medical Support Institutions Model*

Utilization of the location and distribution optimization of medical support institution model are achieved through the systematic model, mainly for the application of the model to the relatively mature field medicine warehouse.

7.4.2.1 Case Scenarios of the Location and Distribution of Medical Support Institutions

When an attack occurs in a combat area, due to the demand for drugs from medical support institutions, a field medicine warehouse in the region is expected to meet the needs for different drugs from support institutions. The latitude and longitude range for the general area of the site is (116.25, 36.33) to (118.51, 34.40).

The Configuration of Medical Rescue Institutions

At present, medical care institutions in the region have been configured for group aid station 1 (118.0247, 36.1307), battalion aid station 1 (118.0450, 35.3113), group aid station 2 (116.5819, 35.5456), group aid station 3 (116.5210, 35.1025), and battalion aid station 2 (117.4733, 35.0440).

The Configuration of the Command Post

The combat logistics command post is set at (117.4048, 35.4811).

The Road Condition of the Main Direction of the Fighting Road

The main direction of the fighting road to a major highway is located on a major road in Jining and Linyi. The road node can be described by latitude and longitude, mainly by five points. The location is as follows: (116.3806, 35.2541), (116.5303, 35.3524), (117.1722, 35.3902), (117.4141, 35.30), and (118.2004, 35.0416).

7.4.2.2 The Optimized Location and Distribution Plan of Medical Rescue Institutions

Pairwise Comparison Matrices of Influencing Factors

Hierarchical structure of the field medicinal warehouse and pairwise comparison matrices of various factors can be established via expert consultation. The factors beneficial to medical supply include the following: near the main direction of the road, near the railroad terminal, near the command post, and near major highways. The factors beneficial to medical safety include the following: easy to be hidden, away from rivers, and avoiding major military targets and low-lying land (Table 7.1).

Weight Values of Influencing Factors

By setting parameters of the locations, we can generate a field medicine warehouse location after determining the optimal solution. The difference between the location of the minimum unit is fixed to 30 s of latitude and longitude, among which the main factor is the weight value caused by location and distribution input. Thus, the number of quantitative indicators can be quantified, while for some qualitative indicators, such as being easy to be hidden and avoiding low-lying land, among others, we can obtain information directly from the map (Table 7.2).

The Optimal Solution of the Location of the Field Medicine Warehouse

After determining the quantitative indicators, we can run the model to calculate the weight values of factors influencing locations and obtain the smallest unit of the comprehensive weight values of various locations via GIS. According to the given conditions of medical rescue institutions, the command post, and the configuration of the main direction of the road, the optimal situation is located at (117.1030, 36.4000), with a comprehensive weight value of 0.24, and the subtotal of its distance to all medical rescue institutions is 16.09 km (Table 7.2).

7.4.2.3 Distribution Optimization of Medical Institutions in Regional Forces

An Overview of Distribution of Medical Institution in Regional Forces

Distribution of Healthcare-Secured Population

War zone XXX is comprised of XXX units, scattered over 137 regions that are above the county level, with a total population of XXX. Subsection A answers to XXX units while subsections B and C safeguard XXX units and XXX units,

Table 7.2 The quantitative indicators influencing the location of field medicine warehouse

Factor categories	Quantitative indicators (miles)
Near the main attack road	5
Near the command post	5
Near the railroad terminal	6
Near the major highways	8
Away from rivers	5
Avoiding major military targets	5

respectively. The geographical distribution pattern unveils an uneven distribution of regional forces with a higher density of urban and coastal population and a sporadic pattern in remote areas. In general, the distribution patterns of healthcare-secured people in S province and H province bear resemblance. By administrative division, subsection C has a larger population (accounting for almost half of the total population), while a smaller population is equally shared by subsections A and B.

Distribution of Military Medical Institutions

This war zone exists across X provinces with XXX basic medical evacuation teams and three logistics subsections (A, B, and C). XXX military hospitals are allocated to this war zone including X general hospitals, X central hospitals, and XX division hospitals. XXX beds are originally designed, among which XXX are actually in use.

XX military hospitals are located in this war zone, dispersed across 21 cities. Subsection C possesses the most hospitals (XX), while subsections B and A accommodate fewer hospitals with a similar quantity.

Judging from the geographical distribution pattern, military hospitals in this entire war zone are sensibly established in that basic medical evacuation is secured. However, in some large- or medium-sized cities, resources are excessively allocated and beds are intensively provided. C13 and A1 are both unnecessarily privileged, with two hospitals with H13 and H14 in C13 and H0 and H1 in A1.

From the perspective of systems division, the medical systems within the area are poorly marked out. For instance, Unit 171 is less than 10 km from H17, but the designated hospital is H14, which is 65 km away. Unit 173 falls into the 10-km radius with H21 as the center, while the designated hospital is also unreasonably set as H14.

Analysis of Medical Security Relations in Regional Forces

Parameters

(i) *Effective service radius of military hospitals*

In accordance with the Regulations of Medical Institutions and Guidelines on Establishing and Managing Medical Institutions issued by the State Council, along with various characteristics of medical service demand coming from different levels within the army forces and preliminary research results of the project, any hospital above the central level is defined as a large general hospital, while divisional hospitals are considered small general hospitals. In a hypothetical scenario, the effective evacuation time to divisional hospitals and central hospitals is 2 and 4 h, respectively, and the average ideal speed of evacuation vehicles in urban and suburban areas is 25–45 km/h. Based on the formula, Radius = Velocity × Effective Evacuation Time, the ESR of divisional hospitals and central hospitals is 50–90 km and 100–180 km, respectively. In this project, we adopt different schemes and models by presuming 50, 75, and 90 km as the hypothetical ESRs of divisional hospitals and 100, 140, and

180 km for central hospital. Further, we determine the distribution pattern as well as the optimal result.

As illustrated in the figure above, the maximum distance between central hospitals within this war zone is more than 300 km, and the minimum distance is less than 20 km with an average of 130 km. The maximum distance between divisional hospitals is more than 200 km and the minimum distance is less than 40 km with an average of 100 km. Central hospitals are, on average, 120 km away from divisional hospitals (7.4). Subsection B accommodates two central hospitals and four divisional hospitals, with 40–130 km of distance between hospitals of the same military level and 70–120 km of distance between cross-level hospitals. Subsection A has four hospitals of central level or above and three divisional hospitals. H0 and H1 are within a 20-km perimeter. Therefore, the distribution pattern of military hospitals in this section is poorly designed. A smaller number of central hospitals in close proximity are located in subsection C, which holds only two central institutions and eight divisional ones.

After referring to previous information, consulting with specialists, and accounting for the relations between hospitals of different military levels, this project sets the ESR of divisional hospitals as 50 km and that of central hospitals as 100 km. The major task for military hospitals within the war zone is to admit the injured from upper-level hospitals and provide them with treatment and care. However, considering the limited number of H0 in the war zone and the fact that H0 does not act as a security force that directly performs medical care, optimization on H0 will not be carried out in this model.

(ii) *Medical Service Capacity of Military Hospitals*

In view of the utility rate of bed resources, demand of military medical service, and the expected functions and tasks of military hospitals, we set the capacity of each bed in central hospitals as 150 patients and divisional hospitals as 120 patients. The overall capacity of military hospitals of different levels within the warzone, after calculation, is demonstrated in Table 7.3.

Analysis of Medical Service Security Relations

By combining the geographical distribution pattern of the military hospitals and garrisons and the ESR calibrated in the previous section, we can establish a distance matrix, whose function is to determine whether military hospitals fall into the parameter.

(i) Based on all the factors, such as geographical location of subjects and effective medical service radius, we establish a coefficient matrix under constraint conditions in order to calculate the distance between troops and military hospitals and further determine the interconnections. From the measurement, the maxi-

Table 7.3 Military hospital capacity in war zone XXX

Military hospitals	Total beds	Capacity
Central hospital		
H15	250	37,500
H13	500	75,000
H2	350	52,500
H3	250	37,500
H7	360	54,000
H10	250	29,250
H1	250	29,250
Divisional hospital		
H16	200	23,400
H19	250	29,250
H20	100	11,700
H21	100	11,700
H18	150	17,550
H22	100	11,700
II17	200	23,400
H14	300	35,100
H6	100	11,700
H5	100	11,700
H4	200	23,400
H9	100	11,700
H12	100	11,700
H11	100	11,700
H8	200	23,400

mum distance between troops and the closest military hospital is more than 200 km and the minimum distance is less than 10 km. Among XXX troops, 85.70 % are located within the effective radius of XX hospitals. When it comes to subsections, the percentage of troops located within the parameter in subsections A and B is 97 % and 88 %, respectively, as subsection A has a larger number of central hospitals and thus has a wider effective service zone. As subsection C answers to a more extensive area with a larger population, 28 % of the troops are not within the effective service zone.

(ii) Medical service relations could be optimized by models under the principle of service troop allocation. The optimization plan is shown in Table 7.4. H19 answers to the most military hospitals in the war zone, whose treatment quota reduces from 26 hospitals to 19 after optimization. Apart from H0, H9 provides medical service to only four troops before the application of the optimization plan, and it also answers to the fewest hospitals along with H8, which is responsible for only four hospitals. H7 has the largest capacity, with a treatment quota that expands from 47,365 to 49,474 patients, while H9's capacity is the least desirable, with a quota that drops from 10,804 to 7201 patients after optimiza-

Table 7.4 Optimization plan

Hospital	Number of beds	Before		After	
		Unit	Capacity	Unit	Capacity
H0	600	2	11,149	2	11,149
H2	250	8	18,845	6	16,055
H7	250	15	47,365	14	49,474
H3	250	10	17,920	12	16,845
H12	150	13	21,397	10	13,851
H10	250	6	24,600	8	33,880
H15	250	6	19,525	12	33,558
H13	500	6	22,803	17	56,643
H6	250	13	17,564	11	13,443
H5	100	9	16,560	9	15,090
H4	130	9	16,793	7	14,299
H9	80	4	10,804	4	7201
H12	100	9	18,879	12	26,673
H8	100	5	34,861	4	32,095
H11	100	7	11,539	6	10,429
H16	120	5	18,485	5	15,713
H19	200	26	32,859	19	20,341
H20	100	14	28,394	14	28,131
H21	100	14	17,700	11	11,430
H18	100	9	24,698	10	18,944
H22	80	7	17,515	5	14,820
H17	100	10	22,892	8	11,026
H14	300	10	25,455	6	24,759
Total	4310	215	504,319	214	495,849

Note: Unit 114, located beyond War Zone A1, is covered by H21 with a capacity of 8470 people. The map is not optimized due to the model constraints

tion. To conclude, medical service capacity witnessed an increase in only four military hospitals, indicating that the medical security system in this war zone is not properly implemented.

Distribution Optimization Plan of Medical Institutions in Regional Forces

Analysis on Capability of Medical Institutions

If we take medical service capacity as the constraint condition of the model, one central hospital (H7) and seven divisional hospitals (H16, H20, H18, H22, H5, H12, and H8) are overburdened with excessive workload within the war zone after optimization. Compared to conditions prior to optimization, the workload of all hospitals (except H12) decreases, and each divisional hospital is equipped with 100 beds. The overload can be accounted for by intensively distributed systematic troops, the small size of military hospitals, and the discrepancy between hospital size and assignment, which could be addressed by adjusting the scale of hospitals.

Analysis of Distance from Operation Sites

Before optimization, the add-up distance between XX systematic troops and XX military hospitals is 19,830 km, and the average distance is 46.50 km. After the improvement model is introduced, the overall distance is reduced to 17,500 km with an average distance 45 km. Optimization resulted in 2330 km of reduction in add-up distance and 1.5 km of cut-down in average distance between a troop and its corresponding hospital.

All systematic troops that are affiliated with medical support institutions have witnessed changes in the process of optimization, and 51 changes are introduced in security relations within the war zone. Before the optimization, 46 systematic troops were beyond the parameter of the divisional hospital's effective service, that is, the original evacuation distance of these 46 troops is more than 50 km, and they account for 90.20 % of all troops in the war zone. The average evacuation distance is shortened by 13 km after optimization from 65 km to 52 km.

Distribution Optimization of Medicine Supply Institutions in Regional Joint Service Forces

Based on relevant statistics from medicine supply institutions in war zone XXX as well as from military medical institutions above regiment level, we attempt to adjust and improve medicine supply security relations in this area.

Overview of the Distribution of Medicine Supply Institutions in Joint Service Forces

After systematic adjustment, the war zone is divided into two sections: subsections A and C. The major medicine supply institutions within the war zone are G001, G002, G003, and G004, with the former three affiliated with subsection A and G004 affiliated with subsection C. These four institutions are situated in two provinces. Given the geographical layout, G001 and G002 are the closest to each other, in terms of medicine supply security.

Medical institutions and management faculties above regiment level amount to XX, covering XXX people in total. Subsection A has a marked advantage over subsection C in terms of the number of people under supply. G001 has the most supply units, while G004 covers the most people. Given the distribution pattern, G004 is located inland where regional troops are intensively distributed, while G003 resides in the coastal area where the distribution intensity of regional forces is more prominent than the other three institutions. In comparison, troops in G002 are sporadically located.

Analysis of Medicine Supply Security Relations in Joint Service Forces

The overall distance between four medicine supply institutions and their corresponding units reflects various degrees of delivery complexity. As shown in the figure, the length of different routes varies.

The overall distance from G002 reaches 13,819 km, with an average distance 288 km. However, the supply capability of G002 is the weakest, and G002 is comparatively distant from receivers. Therefore, it will undoubtedly result in a higher cost in the process of delivery, which is against the principle of high efficacy and low costs.

Distribution Optimization Plan of Medicine Supply Institutions in Joint Service Forces

Analysis on Capability of Medicine Supply Institutions

After optimization, the supply channels of 58 medical institutions above regiment level saw changes within the war zone, with G002 witnessing the most dramatic change whose medicine supply institutions increased to 22. G002 was originally responsible for 33 institutions, but 30 of them were overtaken by G004 after optimization. Most medicine supply institutions affiliated with G002 are beyond its security zone. They are either in the area of G004 or actually in the zone. Therefore, security relations before optimization fail to follow the principle of closeness and convenience. It is also noteworthy that G003 and G004 have a wider supply channel after optimization. G001 was originally responsible for 25 institutions, but 18 of them were undertaken by G003 after the application of the plan.

Prior to optimization, it was beyond G002's financial capability to answer to the expected population, while the potential of G003 and G004 had not yet been fully realized. Under the post-optimization condition, the duties of G002 are markedly reduced, more or less equivalent to its capacity, while G003 and G004 became strained and overloaded. In comparison, G001, as specialized medicine storage, is capable of supplying more. Therefore, in light of the geographical position of G002 and its changes after optimization, we propose a moderate reduction of the size of G002 and the transfer of some supply targets to G001. This will reduce the burden of G002 and make full use of G001's resources. In addition, a moderate expansion of the scale and capacity of G003 and G004 is suggested.

Analysis on Distance from Operation Sites

After optimization, the add-up distance between the medicine supply institutions and targets reaches 23,741 km. The distance of each institution from operation sites, along with the average distance, is displayed as below.

Only the maximum distance of G004 is prolonged after optimization, while six of its additional supply targets are more than 250 km away from institutions, which is an objective result of subsection C's comparatively larger security zone. This also stresses the necessity of actualizing joint service forces. If possible, we could forego boundaries between war zones and assign T115, T129, T043, T003, T108, T033, T166, and T067, which are distant from G004, to the other security zone in accordance with the proximity principle so that the maximum distance could be shortened, thereby improving security efficacy.

References

Abolghasemi H, Poorheidari G, Mehrabi A, et al. Iranian military forces in the Bam earthquake [J]. Mil Med. 2005;170(10):859–61.

Amundson D, Lane D, Ferrara E. Operation aftershock: the U.S. Military disaster response to the Yogyakarta earthquake May through june 2006. Mil Med. 2008;173(3):236–40.

Baker MS. Creating order from chaos: part I: triage, initial care, and tactical considerations in mass casualty and disaster response. Mil Med. 2007;172(3):232–6.

Kang P, Zhang L, Liang W, Zhu Z, Liu Y, Xu L, Yang H. Medical evacuation management and clinical characteristics of 3,255 inpatients after the 2010 Yushu earthquake in China. J Trauma Acute Care Surg. 2012;72(6):1626–33.

Lulu Z, Xu L, Youping L, Yuan L, Zhipeng L, Lin J, Shen J, Xuefeng T, Yi Z, Liang W. Emergency medical rescue efforts after a major earthquake: lessons from the 2008 Wenchuan earthquake. Lancet. 2012;379(9818):853–61.

Ofer M, Nachman A, Gad L, Schwaber MJ, Yitshak K. The Israeli field hospital in Haiti--ethical dilemmas in early disaster response. N Engl J Med. 2010;362(11):198.

Zhang L, Yuan L, Xu L, Yi Z. Rescue efforts management and characteristics of casualties of the Wenchuan earthquake in China. Emerg Med J. 2010;28(7):618–22.

Chapter 8
Modeling Hospital Transition from Peacetime to Wartime

Meina Li, Wenya Yu, and Lulu Zhang

Abstract The research followed the ideology of "evidence-based research" to investigate mechanism of potentiality management, capability development, as well as implementation of civilian hospital mobilization. Referring on complex adaptive system (CAS) modeling theory, the author set up a CHM system dynamics (SD) model with research methods, especially SD modeling technique. With the SD model of CHM system, the behavioral rules were stimulated and analogue simulation of system structure and complicated behavior was realized, thus providing a test platform for relevant policymaking. Then the intervening tests were carried out on the platform to find the intervening target for improving system performance. Policy recommendations proposed to increase the capacity of CHM system provide a theoretical basis for the building of mobilization capacity.

8.1 Introduction

8.1.1 Current Situation and Literature Review

In wartime or in military operations other than war, the armed forces of many countries carry out the health and epidemic prevention work that they perform on the battlefield for civilians in collaboration with local health departments. They recruit civil transportation power for the evacuation of sick and wounded people and mobilize local hospitals and other medical institutions to treat the wounded (Ku and Huang 2005).

M. Li, PhD • W. Yu
Department of Military Health Service, College of Military Health Service,
Second Military Medical University, Yangpu, Shanghai, China

L. Zhang, PhD (✉)
Department of Military Health Service, College of Military Health Service,
Second Military Medical University, Shanghai, China
e-mail: zllrmit@aliyun.com

© Springer Science+Business Media Dordrecht 2016

L. Zhang (ed.), *Modeling the Injury Flow and Treatment after Major Earthquakes*, DOI 10.1007/978-94-017-7527-4_8

8.1.1.1 Local Hospital Mobilization Laws and Regulations

The United States established a systematic and complete statute that is composed of a variety of separate regulations. These regulations cover various fields of preparation for and implementation of local hospital mobilization, including mobilization policy, mobilization preparation, mobilization organization construction, mobilization implementation, and issue mobilization orders. These regulations form a crisscrossed, interconnected, strict, and complete system. This system includes the "National Security Law," "War Authorization Act," "National Emergency," "Armed Forces Reserve Act," "National Defense Production Act," "National Defense Authorization Act," "National Defense Equipment Act," "Trader Law," "Civil Aviation Reserve Regulations," "Wartime Emergency Orders," and so on. (The first three laws on this list are the basic military laws. The next four are higher-level laws.) Among the laws of this system, the "Strategic and Critical Materials Reserve Act," "National Security Law," and "National Defense Production Act" constitute the fundamental code that serves as the basis of war mobilization in the United States (Zhao 2004). The revision of the Selective Military Service not only reemphasized the necessity of having a mobilization plan for the health sectors but also pointed out the substantive issues that need to be solved in the early period of mobilization (Aufranc 1951).

The specific requirements of local hospital mobilization in Britain are contained in civil, administrative, and economic laws. For example, the "Civil Aviation Law" and "Transportation Law" clearly state that the government is entitled to all types of appropriate transportation from nationalized enterprises when there is a national defense need. For private forms of transportation, the government usually signs a "Contract Agreement" in peacetime, but these forms of transportation can be expropriated after an emergency authorization from the Parliament. In the Falklands War, the British completed the modification of hospital ships within 3 days. During the Gulf War, the British Government was the first one to respond to the call for establishing multinational forces. It authorized the Royal Army Medical Reserve to call up a team quickly, and 1500 reservists were conscripted. Many of them were sent to the Gulf to strengthen the medical support for the British forces who were implementing the "Granby military action." The rest were distributed among 14 medical units around the country that had prepared to treat the sick and wounded who returned from the front line. According to the experience of hospital ships in the Falkland War, the British Royal Navy quickly transformed a fleet auxiliary vessel called "Argus" into an ambulance ship with 360 medical and technical personnel as well as 4 Marine Corps helicopters.

The National Association of France issued the "National General Mobilization Act" in 1793, which was the world's first mobilization regulation. France promulgated the "General Mobilization Law" in 1938 as the basis of other mobilization laws, thus forming a complete legal system (Mobilization division of General Staff. CPLA 1992). According to the "National Defense Law," "Civil Defense Law," "National Defense Mobilization Law," "Health Mobilization Law," "Manpower Mobilization Law," and other regulations, the French army could enlist all kinds of personnel to support the front line. In January 1958, the national ministries of France jointly issued instructions detailing how the medical systems of military departments should act together to address crises that might emerge in the shortest time. The "2000 Reserve Plan" of France reclassified reserve personnel and established a professional reserve composed of medical personnel, engineers, and translators that could be requisitioned at any time.

8.1.1.2 Local Hospital Mobilization Agency

In order to be ready for the work of local hospital mobilization during wartime, each country has gradually established relatively sound mobilization institutions, each with their own characteristics and practices. Israel has built a war mobilization committee in peacetime and developed a reserve system. The highest decision-making body that oversees French mobilization is the cabinet council, which takes responsibility for making decisions about total or partial mobilization. The Ministry of Defence in France is the highest-ranked leadership institution that oversees hygienic mobilization work. In World War II, the US military set up the Medical Army Procurement Agency (formerly the Naval Medical Procurement Office) (Kretschmer 1950). The Health Resources Advisory Committee was established in August 1950, and it was appointed by the president to be the National Advisory Committee for the levy of the military service system (Griffith 1995). The Health Resources Advisory Committee is primarily responsible for the following (Miller 1953): the wartime mobilization, allocation, and use of medical staff; providing sanitation services; providing veterinary services and early detection of new diseases that biological weapons may induce; utilizing hospitals, clinics, laboratories, other medical facilities, and appropriate first aid places; providing medical machinery, pharmaceuticals, chemical products, biological products, and blood and blood products; and making suggestions to strengthen the teaching and research of the health field. The United States has established a mobilization organization that regards the Ministry of National Defense as its core and brings together the military departments and the Department of Veterans Affairs. This mobilization organization directly assigns mobilization duties and functions to each department. The United States also set up a committee to prepare for emergency mobilization and war at the end of 1981. It bridged the gap between mobilization policy formulation and the execution of a national emergency mobilization plan and coordinated departments' attempts to solve problems that arose in the process of mobilization. This committee is the highest national mobilization policy coordination mechanism and is under the auspices of the National Security Council (Rowe 2003). So far, the main sectors of the US Congress, government, and military are involved in the mobilization up to more than 80 sub-organizations, in which Congress accounted for 1/3 and military and political systems accounted for 2/3. War mobilization has become a global work in all sectors of society. The National Disaster Medical System of the United States undertakes the task of dispatching medical teams during wartime or disaster time. These teams remove sick and wounded people from disaster areas and work with national hospital networks to provide definitive treatment.

The mobilization agency of China at the national level is the National Defense Mobilization Committee (National Committee of State Action). Its main missions are to implement the military strategy of active defense; organize and implement national defense mobilization; coordinate the relationship between the economy, military, and government; use human and material resources for national defense mobilization; enhance national defense strength; and improve the capability of transitioning from peacetime to wartime. The Health Mobilization Office is under the leadership of the National Defense Mobilization Committee, which is in charge of coordinating national health mobilization proceedings. At the regional level, the People's Governments of military regions and provinces, regions, cities, and counties all set up a corresponding national action committee. Each national action committee had a subordinate economic mobilization office that was separately in charge of health mobilization work (Zhu et al. 2005).

8.1.1.3 Regional Hospital Mobilization Preparation

Each nation has made an effort to improve the accuracy of local hospital mobilization plans through means such as establishing various combat models of potential wars in order to do simulation experiments; formulating plans for production, transportation, and storage; and improving scientific and operational plans through drills (Huang et al. 2008). In order to effectively shorten the war mobilization process and quickly realize the potential level of wartime mobilization, the United States developed a series of mobilization plans for various local hospital mobilization activities. These plans stated that government departments have the duty to implement mobilization within the shortest time (Zhao 2004). Military medical procurement agencies developed a procurement plan about the use of military medical equipment and devices in wartime. These plans included not only the suppliers and sources of raw materials but also the ways to obtain these materials (Kretschmer 1950). The United States also widely used information network technology in the Iraq War in order to accurately predict the amount of supplies needed for the fighting forces. America made full use of a medical automation mobilization system that strove to mobilize supplies in a timely, appropriate manner, provide the right amount of mobilization, and make the cost-efficient ratio of mobilization more scientific (Tao 1995). Britain has formulated wartime medical plans, acquired a wealth of information about health and material resources, and archived this information into computers for management (Zhao 2005).

Medical health workers' skills with crowd control, registration, and tracking; information management; disposal; and emergency trauma treatment, which are crucial for local hospital mobilization preparation, have improved due to training (Emery et al. 2009; Phlmann et al. 1986). In order to enhance the synergetic rescue capability of healthcare personnel (Grant and Secreti 2007) and to provide an adequate number of medical professionals in wartime, all countries launched medical mobilization training to transition local hospitals from peacetime to wartime functions. The Department of Defense of the United States clearly defines wartime first aid training as a strategic task. It also stipulates that reservists should participate in the same training that active health personnel do. Just as the health workers at the forefront of battles who are responsible for initial treatment are required to undergo medical training, doctors and nurses must undergo emergency medical training and receive specialized courses. The US military also provides training on how to treat war wounds that is targeted for health reservists. Through the fields of military exercises and disaster relief missions, it trains health personnel in how to provide rapid response and rescue under various battlefield conditions (Hayunga et al. 1988; Shatokhin et al. 1976). In addition, the US military has attempted to promote military and civilian collaboration with the help of the selected reserve hospitals training (McKinlay et al. 1987). The US military established a joint health readiness training center in the 1980s and 1990s to provide open courses of treatment for the wounded under field conditions so that military medical staff, nurses, dentists, veterinarians, and medical assistants could be exposed to them. These professionals learned new methods and means for treating the wounded, and they understood how to deal with the medical problems of refugees and how to schedule and manage health resources. The former Soviet Union utilized the health staff initial training classes to train medical personnel reservists so that they could work in the army units, warships, medical service units, and other agencies. The defense forces of West Germany adopted collective training, military exercises, and professional conferences to train military reservists (Tao 1995).

8.1.1.4 Local Hospital Mobilization Pattern

The United States used rear hospitals and medical reservists' mobilization in wartime. A successful example of cooperation between American soldiers and civilians can be seen in the formation of the Red Cross Hospital and medical reserve troops during World War I. The Red Cross Hospital brought together medical reserve units that the army could quickly mobilize and deploy, and it was a supplementary source of medical teams and medical units. At the same time, the Red Cross Hospital was a well-organized, functional unit. The other army reservists were individuals. The rear hospital personnel had worked and trained together, and they all knew each other before the war. This meant that they could start working immediately after being mobilized without going through a lengthy training. The first reserve forces of the US military were the medical reserve. In order to improve the efficiency of military medical institutions, especially when the country was experiencing an emergency, the United States set up a medical reserve in 1908 (Currie 1908). The formation of a medical reserve helped the country avoid repeating the chaos and disorder of the medical mobilization in the war between the United States and Spain in 1898 (Charles et al. 1923). After World War II, the Army Reserve Act, which reorganized the reserve, was issued in 1952. Since 1989, the reduction of the US military budget and a higher number of military actions enhanced the importance of the army reserve (Rothberg 1995). The US military medical reserves have unique demographics characteristics. Most medical reservists are male, hold the rank of lieutenant colonel, are over the age of 35, and have a high income (Mangelsdorff 1999). In times of war, medical reservists are called up for active service. Before the Gulf War, the United States estimated that Iraq's chemical and biological weapons for ground combat might bring many casualties to the US military. Therefore, the United States set up 18,500 medical beds in the battlefield and prepared 5500 beds in European and 22,000 beds inside continental United States. During the war in Afghanistan, the United States conscripted tens of thousands of health-based reservists into active service in order to strengthen the protection of combatants. For the recent war in Iraq, the United States employed a large number of medical reservists to the Persian Gulf. The "comfort" hospital ship in the Persian Gulf, the former hospitals stationed in Weymouth, the medical support battalion stationed in Qatar, and the medical wing stationed in Saudi Arabia and Kuwait basically consisted of reserve staff. In the Desert Shield/Storm action, more than 40,000 medical reservists were summoned, 50 % of them were deployed to Southwest Asia and Europe, and 50 % were placed in local military hospitals (Tomich 1991). The reorganization of the military, guard troops, and reserve staff in 1993 meant that reservists were more relied upon for medical and logistical services.

8.1.1.5 Local Hospital Mobilization Means

First, mobilization should be guided by the law. There is a complete system of laws and regulations that deal with foreign mobilization, and it has clear, detailed, and actionable legal regulations and requirements. Therefore, once a war occurs that requires mobilizing health resources of civilian hospitals, it can be implemented quickly and mobilized efficiently in accordance with the law. The US Department of Defense has required that the health support reserve resources of the national disaster medical system be available to use when the needs of national defense mobilization in normal time cannot be met in order to ensure the treatment of the sick and wounded. In the Iraq War, the US military relied on a comprehensive mobilization regulatory system for adequate health service manpower mobilization. It deployed approximately an additional 600 doctors, nurses, and support staff to the Landstuhl Regional Medical Center, which is located in the Landstuhl outskirts of southwest Germany and is the largest US overseas military medical institution. It mobilized two hospital ships—the US Navy T-AH19 "Mercy number" and T-AH20 "Comfortable number"—to move to the Gulf. In the Gulf War, the French immediately mobilized more than 1000 healthcare workers to cooperate with the French army's "fawn" action on the basis of the "General Mobilization Law" and "Manpower Mobilization Law." It also mobilized two other French military hospital ships bound for the Gulf. Second, economic instruments should be used. The fundamental practices in most Western countries are using economic instruments to buy medical supplies and signing guaranteed contracts with contractors (Han and Chen 2006). Third, it is better to seek the help of allied country for health resources. Some countries, for the sake of meeting the needs of wartime medical support, widely mobilize their country's health forces and also use other countries' power to complete medical rescue tasks.

8.1.1.6 Local Hospital Mobilization Academic Research

In order to perfect the mobilization work of local hospitals, many countries carried out a series of studies that focused on the potential of local hospital mobilization and the response impact factors of the health reserve. The US military also studied the capacity of local hospital mobilization. For example, the University of Pittsburgh School of Public Health, with funding from the Resources Bureau and under the supervision of the US Public Health Service, cooperated with state and local medical societies and other professional institutions. It conducted a pilot study of health workforce demand under an emergency situation (Aufranc 1951). The study investigated physicians in Pittsburgh area in order to estimate the maximum number of patients these doctors could admit in a state of emergency. It also investigated the consumption of medical services in this region in order to attain the number of doctors who could be mobilized. Public Health Service implemented another study to determine the amount of mobilization hospitals. These studies helped estimate the minimum number of local hospitals that could be mobilized and determine the amount of health manpower that could be mobilized. The research of Public Health Service about the demand for noncommissioned health officers under a state of emergency provided information about the basic needs of public and nonpublic hospital maintenance for the manpower committee. The 1305 Naval Reserve Hospital of Portsmouth and Grant Medical Center performed collaborative training in local reserve hospitals. This deed was recognized by relevant local and national agencies that believed that this project could provide an opportunity for the medical reserve to gain practical medical technology and the latest medical knowledge, thereby improving the quality of medical reservists' training and their mobilization preparedness (McKinlay et al. 1987). The US Army Research Institute conducted research on how the skills, attitudes, motivations, and fears of health reservists influenced their mobilization response (Dinsdale 2004; Steinbern 1594). Some scholars have conducted investigations to understand more deeply the attitude, readiness, satisfaction, mental health level, mobilization preparation, mobilization, demobilization, and reconstruction of the medical reserve (Mangelsdorff 1999; Nice and Hilton 1992; Stretch et al. 1996). Some scholars have shown with their research that working together with host country doctors can be a rewarding experience for a medical reserve unit (Silverman et al. 1998). Some scholars have studied the health and adaptability of medical reservists (Wynd and Ryan-Wenger 1998). Some scholars have summarized the health staff mobilization experience and health reserve deployment principles (Nolan and Pattillo 1989; Chizh 1995). There are other studies that have proposed replacing medical with civilian staff and establishing a joint military forces medical system (Chizh 1999). All of these studies have provided a reference for developing local hospital mobilization policies and implementing relevant work.

8.1.2 Objective and Significance

8.1.2.1 Objective

Research objective: This research followed the ideology of "evidence-based research" in order to investigate the mechanism of potentiality management, capability development, and the implementation of civilian hospital mobilization. Relying on complex adaptive system (CAS) modeling theory, the author set up a CHM system dynamics (SD) model with research methods, especially the SD modeling technique. With the SD model of CHM system, behavioral rules were stimulated, and an analogue simulation of system structure and complicated behavior was realized, which provided a test platform for relevant policymaking. Intervening tests were carried out on the platform to find the intervening target for improving system performance. Policy recommendations will be proposed to increase the capacity of the CHM system to provide a theoretical basis for building mobilization capacity.

8.1.2.2 Significance

(a) Provide tools for local hospital mobilization decision-making
Making full use of the field investigation data of local medical resources, the author will summarize and comprehensively analyze the potential data, tease out how much important material and manpower can be mobilized, and assess the potential of local hospital mobilization. This research into mobilization potential used Oracle database software in order to store, query, and run statistical analyses of the data and to provide an auxiliary decision-making tool to local hospital mobilization.

(b) Facilitate local hospital mobilization optimization
Through research about the local hospital mobilization mechanism, we provide information about the potential of local hospital mobilization, the elements and means of capacity building, the process of implementing mobilization, the factors that will influence the mobilization effect, and the mobilization operation mechanism. We also can determine the mobilization process, distinguish the tasks of different sectors, and provide a theoretical and practical basis for the optimization and improvement of local hospital mobilization.

(c) Provide an experimental platform for local hospital mobilization policy interventions
Our research depends on the basic assumptions of the complex systems theory of "the system structure and its evolution decision system function." It builds a system dynamics model of local hospital mobilization to provide an effective communication tool for analyzing and learning the structure and characteristics of the local hospital mobilization system. It also provides an experimental platform for developing relevant policies, establishes an SD model simulation in order to obtain the complex system evolution rules and defects of the local hospital mobilization system, and provides policy intervention targets for enhancing the efficiency of local hospital mobilization.

8.2 Data Sources Used in the Model

8.2.1 Collection and Utilization of Existing Data

The following data sources were used in our research model: the demographic data and social economic development data of each index; health statistics of Fujian Province from 2001 to 2005; Jiangxi Statistical Yearbook; China Hospital Yearbook; Chinese Health Statistics Yearbook; data of the pilot work of health mobilization; literature concerning domestic and foreign mobilization policy; and management research detailing the scientific results of domestic local hospitals in recent years.

8.2.2 Data from the Field Survey

According to the needs of topic modeling work, we investigated the basic situation of local hospitals in Fujian and Jiangxi provinces. The aim was to provide a theoretical basis and data support for database construction and to adjust the mobilization system policy of local hospitals.

8.2.3 Data from the Thematic Interviews

In order to understand the comments and suggestions of the relevant units of local hospital mobilization, we interviewed relevant national action committee staff, hospital managers, hospital management experts, and health service experts and listened to their comments and suggestions about local hospital mobilization.

8.2.4 The Summary of the Literature

We consulted related articles in professional journals such as *Military Medicine*, *Armed Forces & Society*, *Disaster Management and Response*, *Southeast China National Defense Medical*, *Military and Economic Research*, *Military Economic College*, *Defense Health Forum*, *Defense*, *National Defense Academic Journal*, *People's Liberation Army Hospital Management Journal*, *Defense Medical Journal of South China,* and *Defense Medical Journal of West-south China.* We also referenced *National Economic Mobilization Guide of China*, *National Economic Mobilization System Modeling and Simulation Research*, *Social System Dynamics*, *System Dynamics*, and other books. We retrieved more than 200 articles on health mobilization, medical reservists, and various kinds of system dynamics modeling.

8.3 Model Construction of Hospital Transition from Peacetime to Wartime

8.3.1 A Conceptual Model of Hospital Transition from Peacetime to Wartime (Fig. 8.1)

Whether the functions of a civilian hospital mobilization system can be effectively carried out depends on the interactions of the government, mobilization agencies, military agencies, and civilian hospitals. The adjustment and optimization of the civilian hospital mobilization system needs to improve the operation mechanism and realize the healthy operation of the system. Therefore, deeper studies about the relationships among the subjects in the system, the system, the external environment, the healthcare needs of the population, the mobilization needs of the military agencies, and the policies of the government and mobilization agencies are needed. These can help analyze the existing problems of the system and achieve the goal of optimizing system performance.

8.3.2 A Logic Model of Hospital Transition from Peacetime to Wartime

There are a variety of complex relationships between the civilian hospital mobilization system and its social environment, and the mutual restrictions, interdependence, and interactions between internal and external factors are also

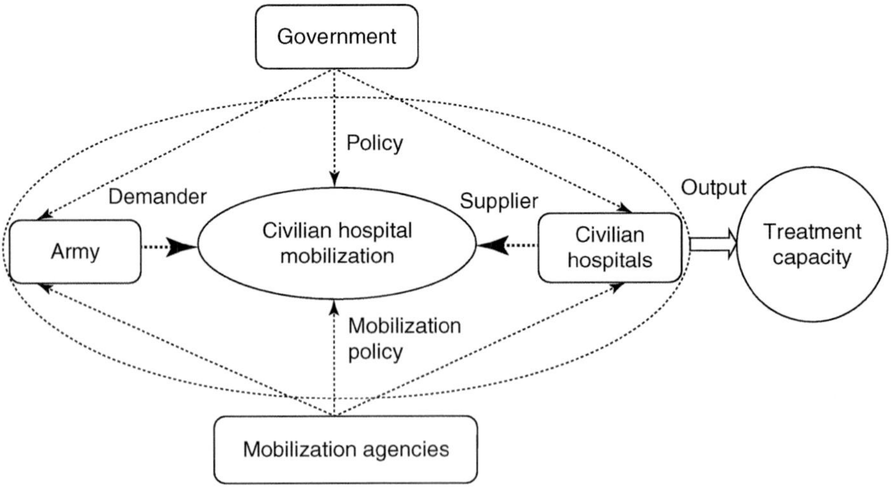

Fig. 8.1 A conceptual model of a civilian hospital mobilization system

important. In this study, the main problem to be solved is the behavioral mechanism, which manages civilian hospital mobilization, builds the organization and command system, and builds the civilian hospital mobilization transition system. We can construct a logic model of a civilian hospital mobilization system through decomposing and synthesizing the results of analyzing the body behaviors and the main loops.

According to a structure analysis of our logic model of a civilian hospital mobilization system, the system impacts the mobilization behaviors of civilian hospitals through government policies and mobilization policies and then feeds back influence to the national security level. The supplier of the civilian hospital mobilization system constitutes the core of the system, and its behaviors interact with the demander of the system, the other subjects, and the external environmental factors of the macroscopic system. The mobilization agency constitutes the periphery of the system, adjusts its behaviors according to government policies and mobilization needs, and is influenced by government policies to a large extent. The analyses of this logic model of a civilian hospital mobilization system illustrate that through the adjustment of the operation mechanism, the system can adjust to the needs of social and economic development, form reinforcing feedback loops of treatment capacity mobilization, rely on the government to develop a complete set of mobilization laws to regulate mobilization and improve the organization management mobilization system, grasp the quality construction of the reserve forces, and realize the structural optimization and sustainable development of the civilian hospital mobilization system.

8.3.3 *SD Model of Hospital Transition from Peacetime to Wartime*

8.3.3.1 Assumptions of a Civilian Hospital Mobilization System

(a) Goals of a civilian hospital mobilization system
The mobilization of civilian hospitals provides an urgent response to the needs of war or the need for treatment capacity in emergencies. Wars and emergencies are characterized by high intensity and fast rhythm, and civilian hospitals are required to mobilize fast and emphasize quality. Therefore, speed and quality are increasingly becoming important standards for measuring the performance of civilian hospital mobilization. Rapid response capability has become an important factor for determining the effectiveness of medical security in wars and emergencies. This study assumes that the goals of a civilian hospital mobilization system are to enhance the response capability of civilian hospital mobilization, to shorten the time it takes to mobilize, to improve mobilization efficiency, and to reduce mobilization costs. In this way, civilian hospital mobilization improves the treatment capacity of war wounds to the fullest extent.

(b) Observation indices of a civilian hospital mobilization system
The main observation indices for this research are completion rate of medical manpower mobilization, per capita cost of mobilization, and the total cost of coordination of manpower mobilization. In order to observe the operation situation of civilian hospital mobilization better, we introduced the completion rate of medical assets and funds mobilization as auxiliary observation indices.

(c) Policy intervention indices of a civilian hospital mobilization system
According to the main causal analysis of the system, the key factors that influenced the speed and quantity of medical manpower mobilization include the potential of civilian hospital mobilization and the capability and preparation of mobilization. Indices are reflected in the following specific ways: the number of medical reservists, the execution rate of organization and command, and the level of compensation for mobilization.

8.3.3.2 Stock and Flow Diagram of a Civilian Hospital Mobilization System

The model of a civilian hospital mobilization system consists of two parts: the organization and command mobilization subsystem and the mobilization activity subsystem.

8.3.3.3 The Main Variables and Functions of a Civilian Hospital Mobilization System

Considering the parameter estimation, we integrated the methods of system dynamics, econometrics, statistics, expert advice, and on-site surveys to identify the key variables. Different types of parameters correspond with different methods and determine the mathematical functions of various equations.

(a) The main variables

I. Level variables
Level variables include the total number of civilian medical personnel, the total number of civilian medical assets, the total number of capitals, the number of medical reservists, the number of medical non-reservists, the total number of medical manpower mobilization, the total number of medical assets mobilization, the total number of capital mobilization, the total cost of coordinating manpower mobilization, the total cost of manpower mobilization, potentiality management, mobilization plans, mobilization orders, the condition of organization and command, and mobilization cost.

II. Rate variables
Rate variables include the increment of medical personnel, the decrease of medical personnel, the decrement of personnel, the increment of non-reservists, the amount of reservist mobilization, the amount of non-reserv-

ist mobilization, the increment of reservists, the increment of medical assets, the depreciation of medical assets, the amount of medical asset mobilization, the total number of cash surplus, and the increment of manpower mobilization cost.

III. Auxiliary variables

Auxiliary variables include the completion rate of medical manpower mobilization, the increase ratio of personnel, the increase rate of personnel, the average personnel expenditure, the parameters of hospitalization manpower, the number of hospitalization, the per capita output of hospitalization, hospitalization incomes, the ratio of supply and demand of hospitalization services, the capabilities of hospitalization services, the rate of medical manpower mobilization, the potential of medical personnel mobilization, the per capita medical output, and the expenditures for medical equipment mobilization.

IV. The initial variables

The initial variables include the per capita annual visits, the proportion of critically ill in a hospital, the average hospitalization price, the performance of the information system, and the initial value of the population.

V. Table functions

Table functions include a chart of the rate of personnel increase, a chart of the rate of medical manpower mobilization, and a chart of the investment rate.

(b) b. Determination of the main function

I. Treatment capacity of mobilization

This study used the classic Cobb-Douglas equation $Y=A\,L^{\alpha}K^{\beta}$ characterization and posited that the discipline of the output growth of civilian hospital mobilization system can be expressed as a function of human resource *L* and capital *K* (Levy et al. 2006). We defined variables in the following manner: *Y* is the system output, indicating the treatment capacity of war wounds; *K* is the total amount of invested capital, expressed as the total amount of medical assets mobilization; *L* is the total amount of system human resources, represented as the total amount of medical manpower mobilization; *A* is the output capacity parameter; and α and β are, respectively, the coefficient of output elasticity of labor *L* and capital *K*, as parameters to be estimated.

Namely, treatment capacity of mobilization = parameters of output capacity of mobilization system * total amount of medical manpower mobilization ^ coefficient of manpower output elasticity * total amount of medical asset mobilization ^ (1-coefficient of manpower output elasticity)

II. Determination of smooth function

A smooth function provides smoothness of information, plays a role in influencing information delay, and is divided into first-order smoothing and third smoothing. A smooth function mainly includes parameters of hospitalization and outpatient manpower.

Parameter of hospitalization manpower = SMOOTH (per capita output of hospitalization/per capita output of medical care/ratio of supply and demand of hospitalization services, TIME STEP * smoothing cycle of manpower allocation)

Among them, "per capita output of hospitalization/output per capita output of medical care/ratio of supply and demand of hospitalization services" is the smooth variable; TIME STEP * smoothing cycle of manpower allocation is the smooth time of variables; and parameter of hospitalization manpower is the smooth value of a first-order index.

Mobilization attractive factor = SMOOTH (average expenditure of mobilized personnel/average expenditure of personnel, Time * 5)

Among them, the "average expenditure of mobilized personnel/average expenditure of personnel" is the smooth variable; TIME STEP * 5 is the smooth time of variables, five steps; and mobilization attractive factor is the smooth value of a first-order index.

III. Determination of logistics delay functions

A delay occurs when quantitative changes need a lag period before their corresponding phenomenon appears, and a delay that occurs in the stream is called a logistics delay (Jia and Ding 2002). For example, medical reservists have to go through a period of mobilization preparation to play their roles, and medical non-reservists need to go through a mobilization preparation time and a training time to learn how to treat war wounds. Therefore, the two variables are both first-order logistics delay functions.

Conversion of reservists = the execution rate of organization and command * whether executing manpower mobilization or not * initiation factor of manpower mobilization * DELAY1 (amount of non-reservists * attractive factor of mobilization, mobilization time, mobilization preparation time)

Conversion of non-reservists = the execution rate of organization and command * whether executing manpower mobilization or not * whether executing non-reservists mobilization or not * initiation factor of manpower mobilization * DELAY1 (amount of non-reservists * rate of medical manpower mobilization * attractive factor of mobilization, mobilization time)

IV. Determination of logic function

Logic function has several types, including MAX, MIN, and IF THEN ELSE. This study mainly applied IF THEN ELSE and MIN logic functions. IF THEN ELSE logic function includes whether executing manpower mobilization or not and the amount of reservists.

Whether executing manpower mobilization or not = IF THEN ELSE (potential of medical personnel mobilization > 0: AND: completion rate of manpower mobilization < 1, 1, 0)

Amount of reservists mobilized = IF THEN ELSE (conversion of reservists < medical reservists, conversion of reservists, medical reservists)

As the number of healthcare service suppliers is not equal to the number of service demanders in reality, we chose the lesser of these numbers as the actual amount of services provided by healthcare agencies through MIN logic function. For example,

The actual hospitalization visits = MIN (amount of hospitalization demand, capability of hospitalization services)

The actual outpatient visits = MIN (capability of outpatient services, amount of outpatient demand)

V. Determination of population function
Based on a literature review and expert consultation, we determined that the amount of population is mainly affected by the birth rate and death rate. According to the theory of system dynamics modeling, we identified the amount of population as an integral variable and thus established the population function.

VI. Determination of table function
Through analyzing the on-site survey data, we initially identified the extreme values and middle values of such variables. Combining them with expert advice, we determined their change trends and thus achieved the chart of increase rate of personnel, the chart of medical manpower mobilization rate, and the chart of investment rate.

VII. Determination of initial values
The initial values referred to in the process of modeling were determined by referencing "Jiangxi Statistics Yearbook 2007," "Chinese Health Statistics Yearbook 2007," "National Campaign Committee of Jiangxi Statistics 2006," and the supplemental data from expert advice and on-site surveys.

8.4 Simulation and Intervention of the Model

8.4.1 Policy Group Screening

In order to observe the influence of changes of system parameters on system behaviors and results, this study designed four groups of intervention trials to observe the system simulation results. Through adjustment of the number of reservists, the preparation condition of organization and command, and the level of compensation for mobilized medical personnel, policy interventions inspired changes to the mobilization time and cost of the whole civilian hospital mobilization system.

8.4.1.1 Adjustment of the Initial Value of Medical Reservists

After increasing the number of medical reservists, we observed whether the adjustment could improve mobilization efficiency, shorten mobilization time, and reduce mobilization cost.

8.4.1.2 Adjustment of the Initial Value of Organization and Command Subsystem

After adjustment of potentiality management, mobilization plans, mobilization orders, and the condition of organization and command, we observed changes to mobilization efficiency, needed time for mobilization tasks, and mobilization cost.

8.4.1.3 Adjusting the Level of Compensation for Mobilized Personnel

After adjusting the level of compensation for mobilized personnel, we observed whether the adjustment could improve the medical personnel's mobilization enthusiasm and shorten the time needed to complete mobilization.

8.4.1.4 Policy Group Intervention Trials

After adjusting the number of medical reservists, the initial value of the organization and command subsystem, and the level of compensation for mobilized personnel, we observed the influence on mobilization times and costs.

8.4.2 Adjusting the Initial Value of Medical Reservists

Current: Initial value of medical reservists is 9300.

Test 1: Initial value of medical reservists is 0.
Test 2: Initial value of medical reservists is 15,000.

The intervention results showed that after increasing the initial value of medical reservists who participated in the civilian hospital mobilization system, the completed time of specific medical personnel mobilization was significantly shortened and vice versa. With an increase of the number of medical reservists, the medical manpower mobilization tasks completed per unit time increased correspondingly, which indicates that the number of medical reservists plays a positive role in promoting the rapid response to civilian hospital mobilization. Among three groups of trials, the per capita mobilization cost of Test 2 was the least, and Test 1 was the most, which illustrates that the form of medical reservists is in favor of controlling the cost of civilian hospital manpower mobilization. According to the results of the three groups, the initial total cost of coordination of manpower mobilization of Test 1 was relatively lower, but with the extension of mobilization time, its total cost exceeded the results of Current and Test 2. The cost of manpower mobilization of Test 2 was always less than the cost of Current. This was due to the fact that the total cost of coordinating mobilization is related with the per capita mobilization cost and the number of mobilized personnel. The rapid response capability of Test 1 was weak, and there were a small number of initial mobilized personnel, even though the per capita mobilization cost was the most. The impact of the number of mobilized personnel led to a lower cost for coordinating mobilization. However, with the progress of mobilization and under circumstances where the number of mobilized personnel was certain, the mobilization cost was mainly affected by the per capita mobilization cost, and this is the moment that reflected the stable trend of mobilization cost, namely, Test 1 > Current > Test 2.

As medical reservists are preparative mobilized personnel and usually are trained systematically, they can respond and mobilize rapidly when civilian health mobilization is needed in wars or emergencies. Obviously, the state of medical personnel in peacetime has an important impact on mobilization, and medical reservists can ensure that mobilization tasks will be completed rapidly and with high quality (Fig. 8.2).

8.4.3 Adjusting the Initial Value of the Organization and Command Subsystem

Current: Initial values of potentiality management, mobilization plans, mobilization orders, and the organization and command subsystem are all 0.2.

Test 1: Initial values of potentiality management, mobilization plans, mobilization orders, and the organization and command subsystem are all 0.0001.

Test 2: Initial values of potentiality management, mobilization plans, mobilization orders, and the organization and command subsystem are all 1.

As shown in Fig. 8.3a, medical manpower mobilization will progress rapidly and be completed in several days when the initial values of potentiality management, mobilization plans, mobilization orders, and the organization and command subsystem are all 1 in Test 2, that is to say, when the mobilization is relatively well prepared in peacetime and the effectiveness of organization and command is fully realized. However, when the initial values are changed to 0.0001 in Test 1, that is, when the mobilization is relatively poorly prepared in peacetime and the effectiveness of organization and command is not fully realized, medical manpower mobilization will progress slowly. During the observation period, only 40 % of manpower mobilization was completed. According to Fig. 8.3b, the per capita mobilization cost in Test 1 was much more than the cost in Current and Test 2. Figure 8.3c separately analyzed the per capita mobilization cost in Current and Test 2, finding that the per capita mobilization cost in Test 2 was always less than the cost in Current. This result illustrated that the more potentiality management, mobilization plans, mobilization orders, and the organization and command are fully prepared during peacetime, the less the per capita mobilization cost will be. Figure 8.3d showed the changes of the total cost of coordination of manpower mobilization, that is, Test1 > Current > Test 2. Figure 8.3e, f showed that if the level of potentiality management, mobilization plans, mobilization orders, and organization and

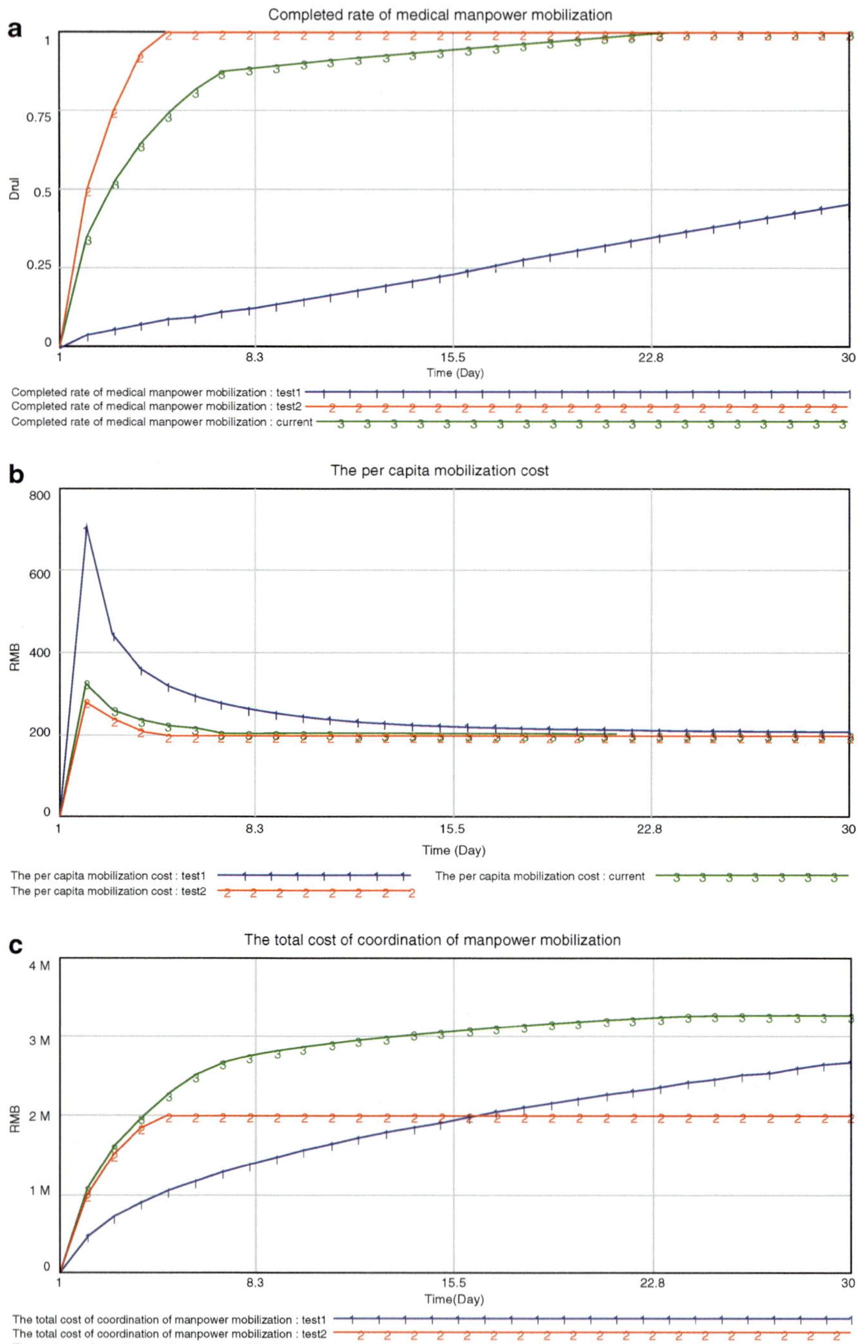

Fig. 8.2 Results of adjusting the initial value of medical reservists. (**a**) Trend change of completed rate of medical manpower mobilization. (**b**) Trend change of the per capita mobilization cost. (**c**) Trend change of the total cost of coordination of manpower mobilization in 30 days. (**d**) Trend change of the total cost of coordination of manpower mobilization in 70 days

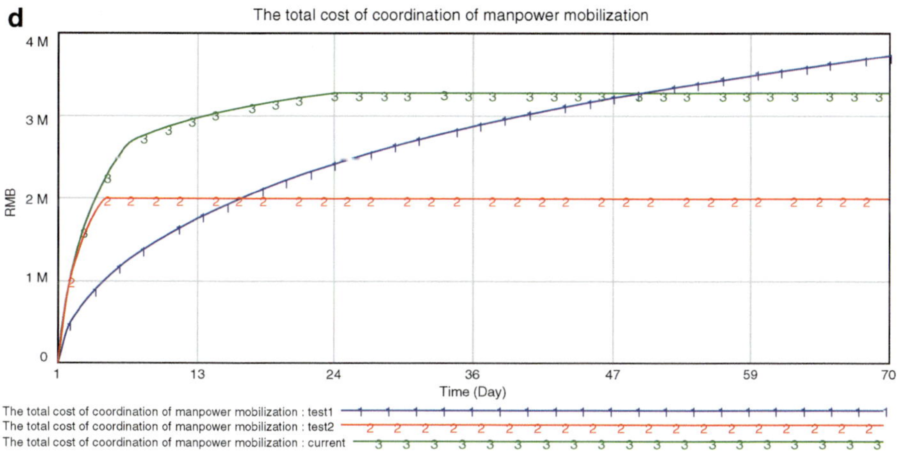

Fig. 8.2 (continued)

command could be improved, the mobilization rate of medical assets and capital would increase dramatically.

Mobilization in civilian hospitals should be based on a certain level of ideology and materials. The more fully the mobilization of organization and command is prepared in peacetime, the more active and reliable the mobilization will be in wartime or emergencies. Therefore, improving the overall effectiveness of the organization and command system is one of the keys to improving the response capability of the civilian hospital mobilization system, and it will help to improve the speed of mobilization and reduce mobilization costs.

8.4.4 Adjusting the Initial Value of the Level of Compensation for Mobilized Personnel

Current: Initial value of the salaries of mobilized personnel is 2 times the initial value of the salaries of medical personnel.

Test 1: Initial value of the salaries of mobilized personnel is equal to the initial value of the salaries of medical personnel.

Test 2: Initial value of the salaries of mobilized personnel is 10 times the initial value of the salaries of medical personnel.

As shown in Fig. 8.4a, when the initial value of the salaries of mobilized personnel was adjusted to 10 times the initial value of the salaries of medical personnel (Test 2), the completed time of mobilization shortened sharply. When the initial value of the salaries of mobilized personnel was adjusted to 1 time the initial value of the salaries of medical personnel (Test 1), the completed time of mobilization increased dramatically. This result indicated that the more compensation for mobilization was provided, the more attractive mobilization was for medical

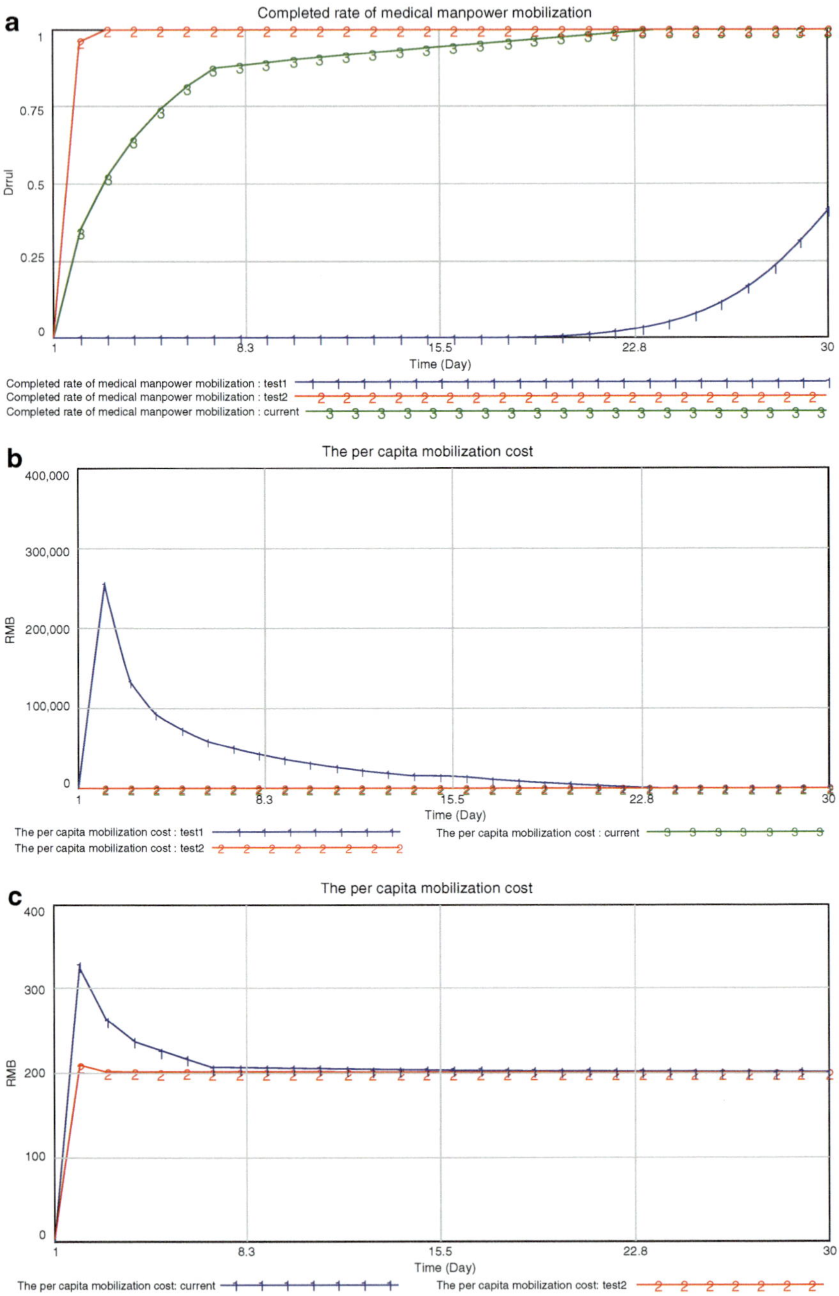

Fig. 8.3 Results of adjusting the initial value of the organization and command subsystem (Tests 1–2). (**a**) Trend change of completed rate of medical manpower mobilization. (**b**) Trend change of the per capita mobilization cost (Test current, Test 1, Test 2). (**c**) Trend change of the per capita mobilization cost (Test current, Test 2). (**d**) Trend change of the total cost of coordination of manpower mobilization. (**e**) Trend change of completed rate of mobilization of medical assets. (**f**) Trend change of completed rate of mobilization of capital

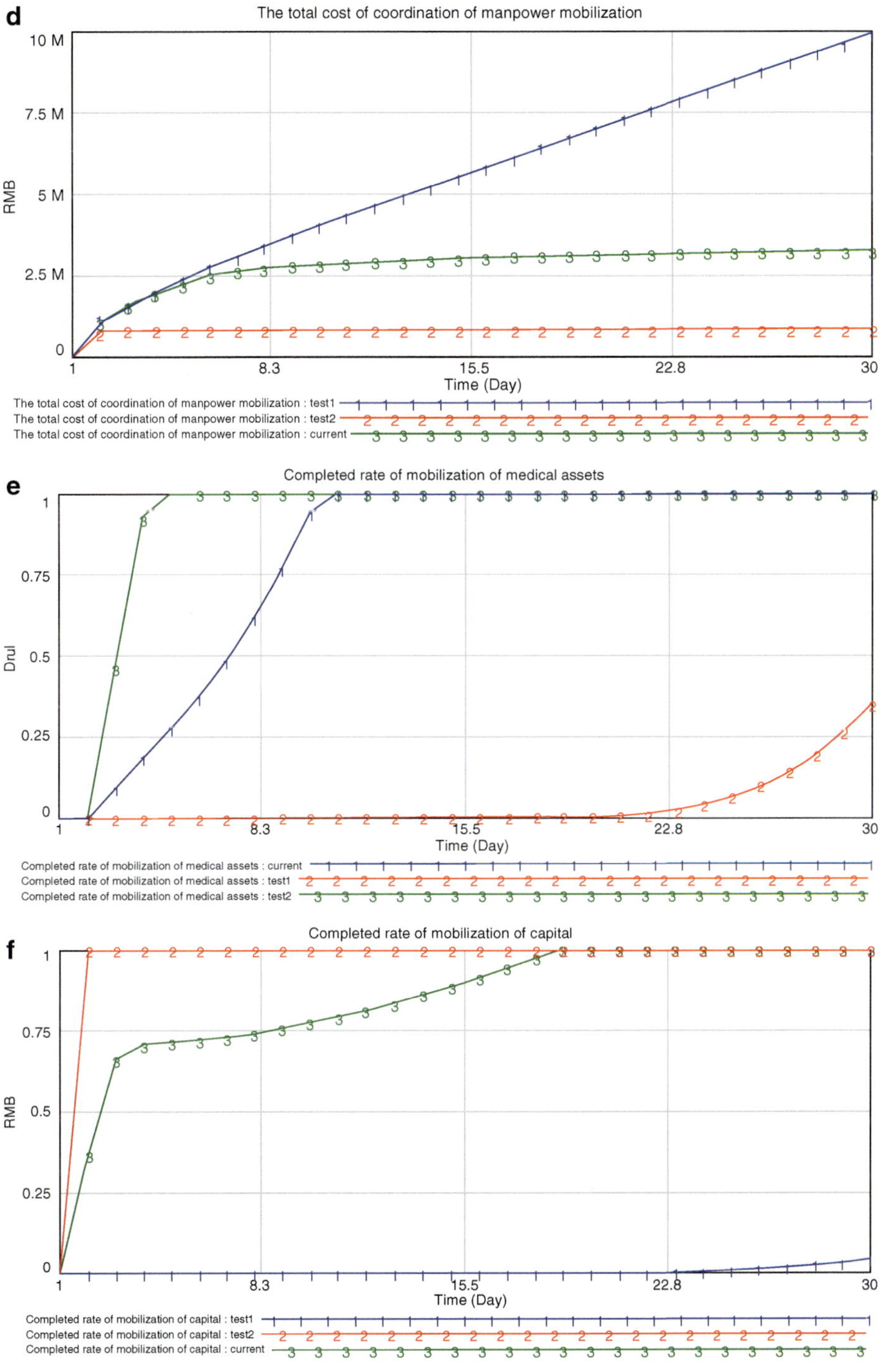

Fig. 8.3 (continued)

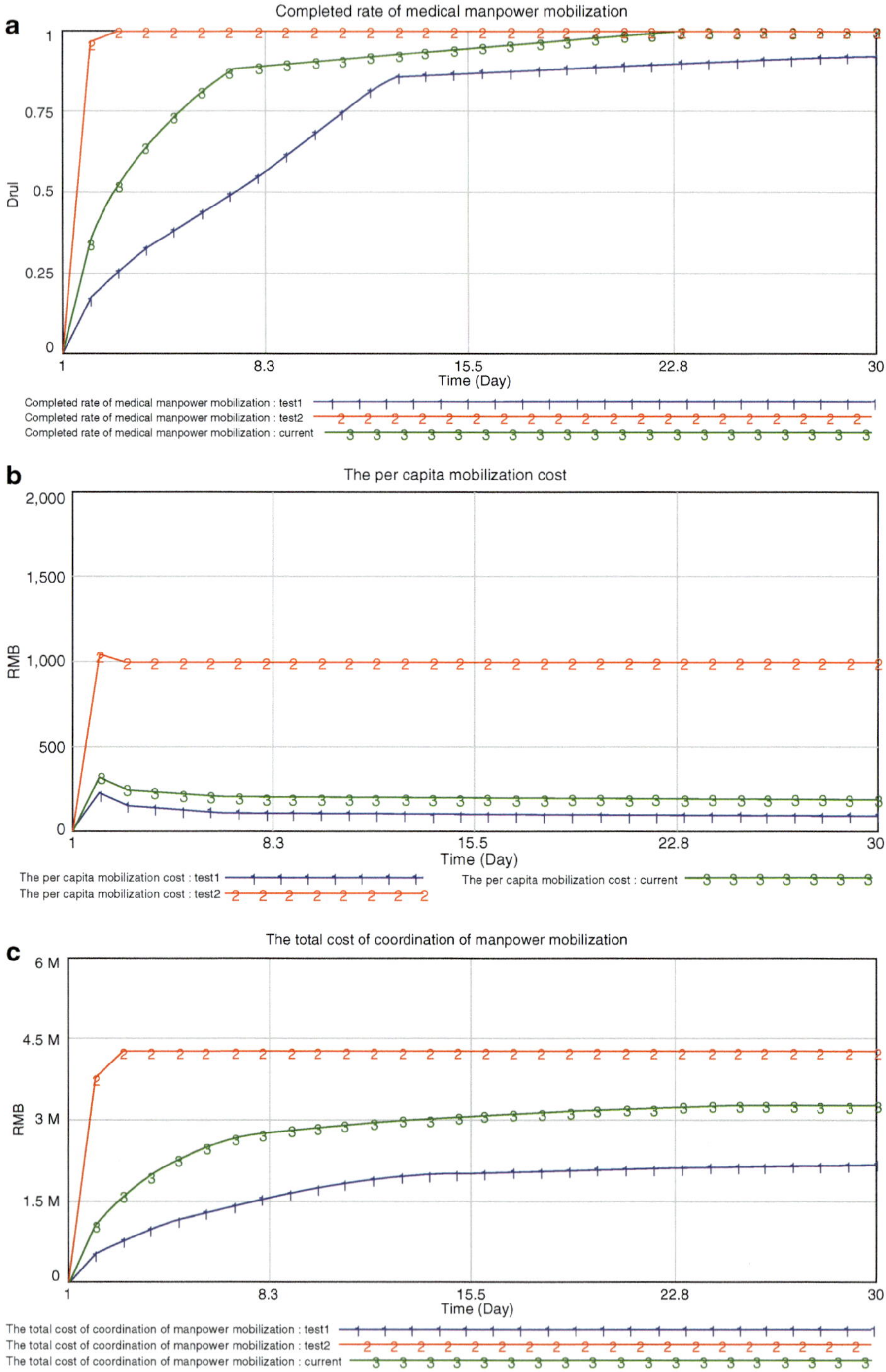

Fig. 8.4 Results of adjusting the level of compensation for mobilized personnel (Tests 1–2). (**a**) Trend change of completed rate of medical manpower mobilization. (**b**) Trend change of the per capita mobilization cost. (**c**) Trend change of the total cost of coordination of manpower mobilization

personnel. The enthusiasm of medical personnel that participated in mobilization greatly improved, and mobilization was completed more smoothly. As shown in Fig. 8.4b, c, improving the salaries of mobilized personnel correspondingly increased the per capita mobilization cost and the total cost of coordinating manpower mobilization. The results showed that improving the level of compensation for mobilized personnel accelerated the process of mobilization and the rapid completion of mobilization but, at the same time, increased the mobilization cost. Thus, when considering mobilization speed and cost, the level of compensation for mobilized personnel should not be too high or too low, and the determination of the compensation level should take into account the national payment capability and the requirements of rapid response to mobilization.

Certainly, the compensation and benefits of mobilization are not only measured by money but also by the credits awarded to medical personnel, the preferential policy of medical agencies, etc. This study quantified these welfare policies in the form of money. It can be seen from the intervention that the condition of compensation for mobilization was also a significant factor that influenced the civilian hospital mobilization system (Fig. 8.4).

8.4.5 Policy Group Intervention Trials

Current: Initial value of medical reservists is 9300; initial values of potentiality management, mobilization plans, mobilization orders, and the organization and command are all 0.2; and initial value of the salaries of mobilized personnel is 2 times the initial value of the salaries of medical personnel.

Test 1: Initial value of the salaries of mobilized personnel is adjusted to 10 times of the initial value of the salaries of medical personnel.
Test 2: Initial value of medical reservists is adjusted to 15,000.
Test 3: Initial values of potentiality management, mobilization plans, mobilization orders, and organization and command are all adjusted to 1.

As shown in Fig. 8.5a, when the initial values of potentiality management, mobilization plans, mobilization orders, and organization and command were all adjusted to 1, the completion of medical manpower mobilization was the fastest. The factors that had a relatively great impact on the speed of medical manpower mobilization were preparation conditions of potentiality management, mobilization plans, and mobilization orders. Organization and command, salaries of mobilized personnel, and the number of medical reservists also improved the mobilization speed. All of the three factors played a positive role in accelerating the mobilization speed. According to the intervention results (Fig. 8.5b, c), improving the salaries of mobilized personnel increased the per capita mobilization cost and the total cost of coordinating manpower mobilization. While improving the number of reservists and the preparation conditions of mobilization reduced the mobilization cost, improving the preparation conditions of mobilization had a more obvious effect on reducing the mobilization cost.

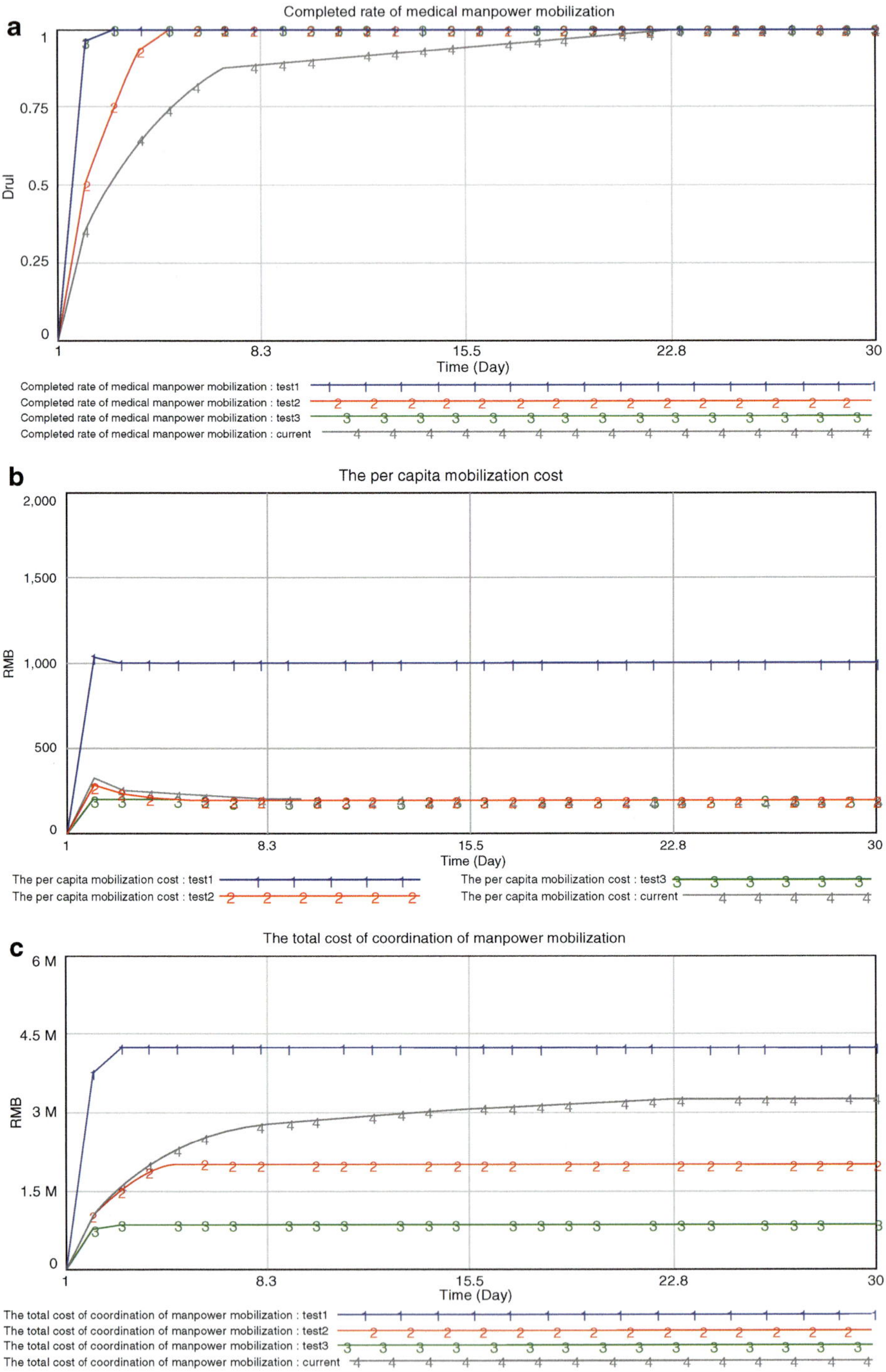

Fig. 8.5 Results of policy group intervention trials (Tests 1–3). (**a**) Trend change of completed rate of medical manpower mobilization . (**b**) Trend change of the per capita mobilization cost. (**c**) Trend change of the total cost of coordination of manpower mobilization

The results showed that preparing mobilization in peacetime helped realize the effectiveness of the organization and command of mobilization system; increasing the number of medical reservists and the salaries of mobilized personnel improved the speed of civilian hospital mobilization; and improving the salaries of mobilized personnel increased the mobilization cost. Therefore, it is better to make policy interventions by adjusting the number of reservists, potentiality management, mobilization plans, mobilization orders, and the organization and command subsystem. Under the circumstances of poor mobilization preparation and low compensation for mobilization, civilian hospitals will evade their obligations of mobilization to some extent, the process of mobilization will be slow, and it will be difficult to complete mobilization in a short time (Fig. 8.5).

8.5 Summary

For civilian hospital mobilization, mobilization speed and mobilization cost are often the key factors. Speed and efficiency are remarkable features of civilian hospital hygiene mobilization, the increase of effective mobilization is largely affected by the mobilization speed, and rapid mobilization has become the main form of hygiene mobilization. In order to complete mobilization in a faster and better way, it is necessary to improve the mobilization speed and control the mobilization cost.

A modest scale of reservists is conducive to the implementation of rapid mobilization. Civilian hospital mobilization should focus on strengthening the connection between mobilization in peacetime and wartime and improving the rapid response capability of mobilization. The medical reservist force is an important force that defends a country in wartime, and it also is an important emergency disposition power needed to complete urgent, difficult, dangerous, and heavy medical treatment tasks and deal with public health emergencies. The term reserve medical support organization mainly refers to the health departments, hospitals, health teams, and independent medical reservist institutions constructed on the basis of civilian medical units according to need (Wu 2001). Educating medical reservists about necessary military medicine, military pharmacy, and military general knowledge in peacetime is beneficial for improving mobilization capacity in peacetime and rapidly forming effective treatment capability during mobilization periods. Planning reserve services is an important move for helping medical personnel in civilian hospitals to closely organize civilian health forces and complete health war preparedness. It is also a significant factor that influences the smooth and efficient completion of mobilization, and it will help to realize rapid mobilization and use civilian hygiene forces (Li 1995). However, the scale of the medical reservist force should not be too large or too small. If the scale of reservists is too large, it will aggravate the national burden. If the scale is too small, the reservists cannot be qualified for missions and tasks. Therefore, the scale of the medical reservist force should be moderate (Wang 2002). Moderation means that national environmental conditions and international status must be adapted to and that various threats to the national needs of medical treatment forces must be dealt with.

Having a sensitive and efficient mobilization command system is a prerequisite for completing medical mobilization tasks. Enhancing the effectiveness of organization and command mobilization is the key to improving the mobilization efficiency in civilian hospitals. Wars and emergencies have strong requirements for mobilization times, and the quality and quantity of mobilization demands can often change in a short time with the changes to external conditions. Relying on mobilization plans and procedures alone cannot guarantee smooth mobilization preparation and implementation. Therefore, it is necessary to improve the capability of mobilization coordination institutions for dealing with various problems arising from mobilization preparation and implementation. According to the medical support needs of future wars or emergencies, we must consider the actual situation of national health undertaking construction; make all systematical, planned, comprehensive, and key preparations for medical mobilization; and improve the organization and command effectiveness of mobilization in civilian hospitals. We should establish a scientific, rational, authoritative, and efficient organization leadership system for civilian hospital mobilization; improve the command institution that can adapt to the requirements of wars and crisis; constantly improve the military and political linkage mechanism; coordinate tightly; interact with supply and demand; and share resources when organizing and implementing mobilization activities. In addition, we should capitalize on the mobilization potential of civilian hospitals, enhance constructions of various medical and health institutions and facilities, improve the level of information and automation of command means, improve plans of civilian hospital mobilization, optimize mobilization plans, and try to make mobilization preparations fuller and more complete in peacetime. This will make mobilizing in wartime or emergencies more active and confident and increase the reliability, sensitivity, and promptness of civilian hospital mobilization (Closer 1994).

The level of compensation for mobilized medical personnel has a relatively great impact on the effect of mobilization. Due to the high education cost invested by medical and health personnel, the returns of the work in which they are engaged are high, and the opportunity costs that they dedicate to the defense cause are correspondingly higher. When countries implement medical manpower mobilization in wartime, mobilized personnel not only have to give up their current jobs and incomes, but they also have to face the danger of death or disability that wars bring. A survey conducted by the US military in 1991 showed that almost all mobilized doctors and ¾ of mobilized nurses suffered economic losses because of mobilization. Medical personnel are reluctant to be mobilized for the following reasons: reduced incomes, lack of respect, family separation, and lack of promotion (Mangelsdorff 1999). Another survey showed that 90 % of medical officers in the air force who have left the army will not join the reservists for fear of having to accept a reduction in revenue at the time of recruitment (Closer 1994). Therefore, when implementing medical manpower mobilization, countries should protect the interests of mobilized personnel by compensating them for the losses they suffer when fulfilling their mobilization obligations. Countries must consider the actual problems of mobilized personnel and compensate them through combinations of direct compensation and indirect compensation, in-kind compensation and value compensation, and material compensation and spirit compensation. In this way, mobilized medical personnel can not only enjoy wages, subsidies, and some basic benefits but have clear benefits and preferential policies in education, further studies, etc. (Liu and Li 2006). If countries can ensure that their incomes and employment status will be protected during their service, solve their worries, and provide appropriate policies to those medical institutions who actively cooperate with defense constructions in peacetime and after wars, the worries of medical personnel and institutions will undoubtedly be solved, medical personnel's enthusiasm about being involved in mobilization would be effectively improved, and conditions for medical personnel to fully safeguard national security interests would be created.

In summary, policy interventions trials of civilian hospital mobilization systems showed that establishing an efficient and sensitive command system for civilian hospital mobilization and a moderate scale of medical reservists and determining a reasonable level of compensation for mobilized personnel will help to improve the speed of civilian hospital mobilization, reduce mobilization cost, and ultimately improve the response capability of civilian hospital mobilization.

References

Aufranc WH. Mobilization of health resources for defense. Radiology. 1951;56(5):641–4.

Charles L, Frank WW, Loy M. The Medical Department of the United States Army in the World War. The Surgeon General's Office. 1923;1:60.

Chizh IM. The organizational principles for the formation of a territorial medical support system for the Armed Forces. Voen Med Zh. 1995;4:18–25. 80.

Chizh IM. Medical support for the Armed Forces: the results and the outlook. Voen Med Zh. 1999;320(1):4–16, 96.

Closer JJ. Challenge of change. The Officer. 1994;70(5):14–7.

Currie JT. Twice the citizen [microform]: a history of the United States Army Reserve, 1908–1995, Currie JT, Crossland RB, editors. Washington, DC: Office of the Chief, Army Reserve; 1997.

Dinsdale P. Medical reservists. The real frontline service. The Health service journal. 2004;114(5928):26-7.

Emery RJ, Sprau DD, Morecook RC, Herbold J. Surge capacity volunteer perspectives on a field training exercise specifically designed to emphasize likely roles during a disaster response. Health Phys. 2009;97(5 Suppl):S155–60.

Grant WD, Secreti L. Joint civilian/national guard mass casualty exercise provides model for preparedness training. Mil Med. 2007;172(8):806–11.

Griffith J. The army reserve soldier in operation desert storm: perceptions of being prepared for mobilization, deployment, and combat. Armed Forces Soc. 1995;21(2):195–215.

Han S, Chen GL. Research on medical reservists rapid mobilization respond system. China J Mod Med. 2006;3(6):26–8.

Hayunga EG, Donaldson PL, Sniffen RA, Holsinger Jr JW. Combat casualty care training for reserve forces. Mil Med. 1988;153(11):574–5.

Huang L, Chen JH, Wu AP. Status and problem of national defense health mobilization. Mil Med J South China. 2008;22(4):77–9.

Jia RA, Ding RH. System dynamics-analysis of feedback dynamic complexity. Beijing: Higher Education Press; 2002.

Kretschmer ET. The mobilization of the medical supply and equipment industry. US Armed Forces Med J. 1950;1(12):1517–26.

Ku GS, Huang CL. New revolution of Military Logistics. Beijing: Peoples Liberation Army Press; 2005.

Levy DT, Bauer JE, Lee HR. Simulation modeling and tobacco control: creating more robust public health policies. Am J Public Health. 2006;96(3):494–8.

Li FR. Exploration of building local reserve hospitals. Mil Med J Southeast China. 1995;S1: 16–8.

Liu HH, Li D. Requirement of military war preparation on national economic mobilization and the strategy. Mil Econ Res. 2006;8:36–8.

Mangelsdorff AD. Reserve components' perceptions and changing roles. Mil Med. 1999;164(10): 715–9.

McKinlay RT, Borden M, Seelig M. Selected reserve-civilian hospital collaborative training: Naval Reserve Naval Hospital Portsmouth 1305 and Grant Medical Center. Mil Med. 1987;152(3):130–2.

Miller SE. Activities of the health resources advisory committee, office of defense mobilization-rusk committee. Am J Public Health. 1953;43(3):322–5.

Mobilization division of General Staff. CPLA. Chinese military encyclopedia-War mobilization. Beijing: Military Science Press; 1992.

Nice DS, Hilton S. Navy Medical Reservists recalled for operation desert storm. Technical report 92–35. San Diego: Navy Health Research Center; 1992.

Nolan DL, Pattillo DA. The Army Medical Department and the Civil War: historical lessons for current medical support. Mil Med. 1989;154(5):265–71.

Phlmann GP, Reynolds Jr NC, Zimmerman RC. Training military reserve medics in combat casualty care: an example of military-civilian collaboration. Mil Med. 1986;151(2):97–100.

Rothberg JM, Koshes RJ, Shanahan JE, Christman KW. Mobilization and rejection of individual ready reserve personnel in operations-desert-shield-storm at a US army quartermaster post. Mil Med. 1995;160(5):240–2.

Rowe JR. Medical support of the Sinai Multinational Force and Observers: an update, 2001. Mil Med. 2003;168(2):110–5.

Shatokhin GV, Ishchenko IK, Mitriakov GR. Military medical training of reserve physicians. Voen Med Zh. 1976;1:21–2.

Silverman MA, Barnes D, Zlamal R, Southworth S, McKinney R, Laubach H, Dileo D, Berger M. Medical readiness training exercise in El Salvador, Central America, 1996. Mil Med. 1998;163(8):519–23.

Steinbern AG. Individual Ready Reserve (IRR) call-up: attitudes, motivation, and concerns. ARI technical research report 1594. Alexandria: US Army Research Institute for the Behavioral and Social Sciences; 1991

Stretch RH, Bliese PD, Marlowe DH, Wright KM, Knudson KH, Hoover CH. Psychological health of gulf war-era military personnel. Mil Med. 1996;161(5):257–61.

Tao MT. Data of foreign military health mobilization外. Military Med J Southeast China. 1995;(s1):46–8.

Tomich N. Medicine in the Gulf War: policy and policymakers. US Med. 1991;27(15, 16):6–11.

Wang FA. Construction of national defense reserve strength. Beijing: Military Science Press; 2002. p. 220–2.

Wu ZY. War mobilization. Beijing: Military Science Press; 2001. p. 177–85.

Wynd CA, Ryan-Wenger NA. The health and physical readiness of army reservists: a current review of the literature and significant research questions. Mil Med. 1998;163(5):283–7.

Zhao XD. National defense mobilization of high-tech regional war of USA. J Nat Defense Univ. 2004;1:95–8.

Zhao YX. Status and mission of health mobilization in China. Mil Med J South China. 2005;19(4):24–33.

Zhu QL, Li HJ, Xie CH. Research of Chinese national economic mobilization. Beijing: Military Science Press; 2005.

Chapter 9
Summary

Yipeng Lv, Chen Xue, and Lulu Zhang

Abstract Through empirical analysis of earthquake emergency medical discoveries, the "two phases" of earthquake casualties and "three stages" of rescue operations are general laws of earthquake emergency medical rescue. Overall, the basic feature was "two phases and three stages," that is, the "growth phase" and "stable phase" of casualties and the "emergency period," "effective segment," and "maintenance period" of rescue operations. Conducting seismic emergency medical rescue organization and command, power organization and management, task switching, and power construction according to relevant laws can help to improve the efficiency of earthquake emergency medical rescue (Lulu et al. 2012). Research on earthquake casualty occurrence patterns is essential for earthquake emergency medical rescue.

9.1 Earthquake Emergency Medical Rescue Complex Model System

9.1.1 The Theory of "Two Periods and Three Phrases"

Through empirical analysis of earthquake emergency medical discoveries, the "two phases" of earthquake casualties and "three stages" of rescue operations are general laws of earthquake emergency medical rescue. Overall, the basic feature was "two phases and three stages," that is, the "growth phase" and "stable phase" of casualties and the "emergency period," "effective segment," and "maintenance period" of rescue operations. Conducting seismic emergency medical rescue organization and command, power organization and management, task switching, and power construction according to relevant laws can help to improve the efficiency of earthquake emergency medical rescue (Lulu et al. 2012). Research on earthquake casualty occurrence patterns is essential for earthquake emergency medical rescue.

Y. Lv • C. Xue
Department of Military Health Service, College of Military Health Service, Second Military Medical University, Yangpu, Shanghai, China

L. Zhang, PhD (✉)
Department of Military Health Service, College of Military Health Service, Second Military Medical University, Shanghai, China
e-mail: zllrmit@aliyun.com

© Springer Science+Business Media Dordrecht 2016
L. Zhang (ed.), *Modeling the Injury Flow and Treatment after Major Earthquakes*, DOI 10.1007/978-94-017-7527-4_9

This book applied numerous modeling methods to deeply analyze the occurrence of earthquake casualties, hospital stay, medical evacuation, medical rescue force allocation, organization and command of earthquake rescue forces, location and distribution of Medical Rescue Institutions, peacetime to wartime in hospital, and so on. This book aimed to determine the intervention targets for earthquake rescue through simulation and modeling intervention, thus effectively improving rescue efficiency and providing a theoretical basis for future rescue capabilities.

9.1.2 Construction of an Earthquake Emergency Medical Rescue Model

This book focused on earthquake emergency medical rescue rules, especially empirical analysis and modeling research. Based on a deep exploration of the earthquake emergency medical rescue field investigation databank, the research group put forward the "two phases and three phrases" theory of rescue system construction. After comparing with domestic and foreign research results, we used several methods used in the health management field, such as system dynamic method, Petri net, and logistic regression analysis and emphasized the construction of the rescue target, logic model connection structure, econometrics model, system dynamic model, multi-agent micro simulation, and so on. With the system view of logic model structure and complex system model integration, the research group established seven key models of health management emergency medical rescue: "casualty flow" and related factors such as "the occurrence of earthquake casualties," "length of stay among hospitalized patients," "medical evacuation in earthquake," "rescue force," and related factors such as "medical rescue force allocation after earthquakes," "organization and command of earthquake rescue forces," "location and distribution of Medical Rescue Institutions," and "from peacetime to wartime in hospital." Further, based on the established models, we conducted a systematic macroscale simulation and intervention experiment to obtain the earthquake emergency medical rescue models, methods, software, and system and provide valuable suggestions for policymakers.

9.2 Results and Suggestions for an Earthquake Emergency Medical Rescue System

9.2.1 Structure of the Emergency Medical Rescue Model

The research group established seven key models of health management emergency medical rescue: "casualty flow" and related factors such as "the occurrence of earthquake casualties," "length of stay among hospitalized patients," "medical evacuation in earthquake," "rescue force," and related factors such as "medical rescue force allocation after earthquakes," "organization and command of earthquake rescue forces," "location and distribution of Medical Rescue Institutions," and "from peacetime to wartime in hospital."

Using the earthquake emergency medical rescue complex model, the research group deeply analyzed the intervention target and key influencing factors and combined domestic and foreign research results to provide a scientific theoretical basis for the development of rescue policy.

9.2.2 *Structure of the Occurrence of Earthquake Casualties Model*

9.2.2.1 Construction of the Occurrences of Earthquake Casualty Model

Earthquake casualties occur at the forefront of earthquake emergency medical rescue. In the previous study of our research group, we used several methods such as the application of mathematical modeling techniques and methods, systems evaluation and qualitative research, descriptive analysis, correlation analysis of statistical methods to compare domestic and earthquake casualty trends, and in-depth analysis of seismic verification of casualties. And we also conducted the review of summarized factors affecting casualties in the Yushu earthquake based on empirical analysis and summarized the strengths and weaknesses of past earthquake prediction model casualties, drawing on casualties for a casualty prediction method using Pareto-simulated earthquake casualties to build a dynamic model for scientific rescue work.

9.2.2.2 Simulation and Intervention of the Earthquake Casualty Occurrence Model

(a) Foreign studies on factors affecting the occurrence of wounded earthquake victims.
   The focal depth of the earthquake itself, the intensity, local geological conditions, and so on will affect the occurrence of wounded individuals, while the local population density and age structure will also affect casualties. Studies on the distribution of casualty locations have come to some conclusions: (1) It is a priority to clear the earthquake situation and the local geological conditions. (2) After the earthquake, most of the wounded are concentrated in the vicinity of collapsed buildings, but not evenly distributed across the affected area. (3) The ability to quickly clear the position of collapsed buildings can effectively reduce waiting time for treatment. (4) The early establishment of geographic information systems (GISs) can play a role in disaster relief.
(b) The prediction trends of the injured being saved every day from the model were in line with the "two-stage" dynamic pattern.

The inflection point came out after the rapid growth period on the sixth day, and the curve entered the stable growth period. After changing the earthquakes' magnitudes, the model's predicting found the following: When the earthquake magnitude was 5, the inflection point was the fourth day after the earthquake, and the first 4 days showed rapid growth in casualties, transitioning to stabile growth after the fourth day. When the magnitude was 6, the inflection point was the seventh day after the earthquake, and for large-scale earthquakes (M8 or M9), the inflection point appeared later (both appearing as the eighth day in the prediction), and the curve is relatively smooth, with a long period of rapid growth and a less-obvious inflection point between the rapid growth period and the stable growth period. This was in line with the earthquake scales' influence on the inflection point of the "two-stage" dynamic pattern.

(c) The model predicts whether arrival of rescue relief in the first 3 days is crucial to reducing casualties.
Therefore, the construction of the local earthquake medical relief forces, as well as the outside medical aid forces arriving in stricken areas within 24 h after earthquakes, could effectively carry out treatment to reduce earthquake casualties, the severity of injuries, and improve the prognosis for the injured.

9.2.3 *Structure of the Length of Stay Among Hospitalized Patients Model*

9.2.3.1 Construction of the Length of Stay Among Hospitalized Patients Model

The ability to identify earthquake patients at risk for longer length of stay (LOS) may be valued by patients and policymakers. LOS, as an important inpatient outcome, has received considerable attention. The current study was undertaken to identify predictors of hospital LOS for patients hospitalized with earthquake-related injury using clinical variables available at the time of admission and hospital characteristics. The present study focused on hospitalized patients from the 2010 Yushu earthquake and comprehensive analyses of medical treatment received by patients. Basing on this situation, we also analyzed the LOS of patients and established an LOS model. The aim of this paper was to identify crucial factors influencing LOS among patients with earthquake-related injury basing on the model established and then to offer insights into directions for effective health policies and clinical pathways formulated to reduce LOS.

A retrospective analysis of 2086 injured victims who were transported from the earthquake area and then admitted to 49 peripheral hospitals (including 8 military hospitals) from April 14 to May 15, 2010, were included in the present study (Kang et al. 2012). Bivariate analysis and stepwise logistic regression were used to explore factors influencing LOS.

9.2.3.2 Result of the Simulation and Intervention of the Length of Stay Among Hospitalized Patients Model

(a) The proportion of males was significantly higher than that of females, and air evacuation played an important role.
The mean (range, SD) LOS was 24.7 (1–203, 18.2) days, and 23 patients (1.1 %) experienced an LOS longer than 3 months. These individuals were generally elderly, female, had bone fractures, or underwent surgery associated with several injury-specific characteristics.
(b) Factors influencing length of stay
Being elderly, female gender, days between injury and admission, bone fractures, injury to the abdomen, injury to the extremities/pelvis, higher injury severity score (ISS), having undergone surgery, and having developed complications were significantly and independently associated with LOS longer than 25 days.

9.2.3.3 Suggestions

Strong preventive and therapeutic initiatives should be designed for elderly and female patients injured in earthquakes, especially within the initial days. Surgery was the greatest risk for a longer LOS. More attention should be paid to patients with fracture, trauma to the abdomen or the extremities/pelvis, complications, and/or higher ISS. The factors identified in this study offer insights into directions for effective health policy to reduce LOS after a devastating earthquake.

9.2.4 Structure of Medical Evacuation After an Earthquake Model

9.2.4.1 Construction of the Model for Medical Evacuation After an Earthquake

Medical evacuation research on earthquake victims mainly indicated that the patients flowed from the disaster area to the rear hospitals for specialized treatment, within the "increasing period," corresponding to the "emergency stage" and the "effective stage." The efficiency of evacuation is directly influenced by structural barriers of the medical evacuation system for patients.

Earthquake medical evacuation system is a complex adaptive system. Guided by the research concept of evidence-informed decision making, we (a) analyzed the orientation, characteristics, mechanism, and principle of earthquake medical evacuation; (b) revealed the subjects' behavior characteristics and rule of system evolution for an earthquake medical evacuation system; (c) built a logic model and SD model of earthquake medical evacuation system; and (d) via the simulation and policy intervention experiment, determined the root of the system structure barriers and function mechanism and put forward policy suggestions to solve the problems of system structure. The research results may assist earthquake relief emergency medical rescue decision making and provide quantitative evidence for earthquake medical evacuation planning.

9.2.4.2 Result of Simulation and Intervention of the Model for Medical Evacuation After Earthquakes

(a) Evacuation speed and resource utilization are often the key factors in earthquake relief and medical evacuation.

Speed and efficiency are significant characteristics of medical evacuation for earthquake relief. Evacuation speed of the sick and wounded greatly affects medical evacuation growth, and hence, rapid evacuation has become the main form of disaster medical rescue. In order to make the medical evacuation for earthquake relief faster and better, it is necessary to improve evacuation speed and medical resource utilization. A highly sensitive disaster relief emergency commanding system is a precondition for completing disaster relief medical evacuation. The key to enhance medical evacuation efficiency for earthquake relief is to increase the efficiency of the emergency medical rescue organization and command.

Emergency medical rescue coordination agencies should improve their ability to deal with all kinds of problems in medical evacuation preparation and implementation. Comprehensive and focused preparation of earthquake disaster emergency medical relief should be organized and planned according the needs of earthquake-prone areas and the reality of the local health delivery system, so as to improve the commanding efficiency of medical evacuation (Lulu et al. 2012).

At the same time, a unified commanding organization by military, police, and the public is also needed. An improving linkage mechanism is required to enhance tight cooperation, the interaction of supply and demand, and the share of resources. Improving the level of informatization and automation of command means and perfecting the medical evacuation plan and optimizing evacuation plan are necessary factors. Emergency medical relief after earthquakes could be increased in terms of initiative and confidence. Higher pertinence, dynamics, and promptness would be achieved if a more sufficient and completed preparation is ready in the standard time.

(b) Early evacuation of the sick and wounded is beneficial to shorten the time from injury to specialized treatment, improving treatment effects.

Evacuating the sick and wounded to receive specialist treatment in rear hospitals has become a major avenue to disaster emergency rescue. Early evacuation, specialist treatment, and rehabilitation are new trends in emergency medical rescue of massive casualty incidents.

(c) Proper evacuation ratio of the sick and wounded has an important impact on improving medical evacuation system resource utilization and effectively executing classification treatment.

Proper evacuation ratio, judging from damage range, available medical forces in disaster area, carrying capacity of evacuation carriers, and treatment needs, is a key in improving the resource allocation efficiency of the medical evacuation system and effectively executing classification treatment. It is only by refining the standard of evacuation that adjusting the evacuation ratio according to the distribution of medical evacuation resources can rationalize the evacuation of the sick and wounded and promote effective utilization of medical resources.

(d) Rational allocation of medical forces in disaster-stricken areas and rear hospital resources is key to improve system efficiency of earthquake relief MES.

Medical rescue commanders and team members agree that the 24 h after an earthquake is a key period of medical rescue, and 8 h following the earthquake is a critical period for saving lives. Specialists play a key role in the 72 h following an earthquake and may be withdrawn after this period. Medical forces should make their rounds as early as possible. Specialists could take turns as supplements. Continuous medical needs in evacuation must be considered in choosing rear hospitals. According to our research and literature review, the amount of the sick and wounded people peak in 1 week and last for 2 weeks in most cases. Further, the average length of stay of the sick and wounded following earthquakes is longer, which is likely related to nonmedical causes, such as post-earthquake arrangement. Commanding institutions should thoroughly assess the occupancy load when selecting rear hospitals. Rear hospitals should enhance their emergency management, properly arrange treatment for the sick and wounded, and estimate the need for rehabilitation and mental intervention.

9.2.5 Structure of the Medical Rescue Force Allocation After Earthquakes Model

9.2.5.1 Construction of the Medical Rescue Force Allocation in Earthquakes Model

Earthquake emergency medical rescue forces are the structural foundation of earthquake emergency medical rescue capabilities, and scientific and rational deployment of rescue forces, timely adjustment of the deployment of rescue forces, and implementation of rescue mission conversion are directly related to the efficiency and even the success of the emergency medical rescue. The deployment of earthquake medical rescue forces is conducted according to the complex adaptive systems (CAS) theory, using methods like systems analysis, literature meta-induction, and multi-body modeling, through the retrospective analysis of earthquake emergency medical rescue domestically and abroad. Systematic analyses were conducted on deployment of earthquake medical rescue forces, a multi-agent system model of the deployment of earthquake medical rescue forces was established, and the relationship among the bodies of forces, decision making, and the object in earthquake medical rescue was explored. Through empirical analyses, the efficiency and results analyses of the deployment of medical rescue forces in the Wenchuan and Yushu earthquakes, we determined the rules of deployment of earthquake medical rescue forces (Kang et al. 2012; Zhang et al. 2010).

This section focused on complex problems of the deployment of earthquake medical rescue forces. Based on the defined studies on deployment of medical rescue forces and systematic analyses of deployment of medical rescue forces from a multi-agent perspective, this study formed a research idea of the deployment of medical rescue forces based on multi-agent systems. Moreover, through the main concept models and multi-agent interaction models of the deployment of earthquake medical rescue forces, this section empirically analyzed deployment of Wenchuan and Yushu earthquake medical rescue forces and determined the laws, characteristics, and system evolution process (Liu et al. 2009; Xiang et al. 2009).

9.2.5.2 Results of the Medical Rescue Force Allocation in Earthquake Model

(a) Consistent with basic principles of utilization of emergency medical rescue forces, actualize the module of force utilization during the entire process.

Under emergency conditions, the utilization of emergency medical rescue forces should be based on emergency health needs and intentions of emergency rescue command institutions and combine the terrain and road conditions, epidemiology characteristics, and other medical geography to analyze the development trend of events. Based on this objective reality, the following principles should be considered. First, act in accordance with the emergency conditions and meet the requirements of emergency medical rescue. It should benefit the on-site first aid of the sick and wounded, and the rapid elimination and effective control of the consequences of events. Second, form an efficient emergency medical rescue system. Normally, it should be in accordance with different regions, points, lines, and planes, and the different forces clustering allocation, thus realizing the combination of the local forces in the affected areas, regional supporting forces, and strategic supporting forces; the combination of regional allocation and linear allocation; the combination of prevention, treatment, and evacuation forces; and preventing disjointing of medical evacuation and health and epidemic prevention, as well as avoiding overlapping forces at the same time. Third, adapt to the objective conditions of roads and traffic. It should be close to the main roads, have enough land and corresponding water, and be close to other rescue forces, thereby facilitating emergency medical rescue for the other rescue forces. Meanwhile, it should strive to avoid possible natural disasters or spreading locations, such as floods, landslides, and downwind direction of nuclear and chemical accidents. The mobile emergency medical rescue forces must follow the function modules, the elements and types of service preparation should be well appointed, and they must adapt the method of module allocation during the entire process. Combined with different mission requirements and in accordance with the module allocation requirements, it is necessary to establish treatment function modules to adapt to different geographical, natural, and technical conditions. It should strengthen the construction of the components of medical treatment function modules and the construction of the structure standards and promote the conversion of resources to security forces. Meanwhile, it requires improving types of functional element modules, equipped with the necessary professional rescue modules, including obstetrics and gynecology, pediatrics, and psychology, thus realizing a professional module with multiple functions as well as good mobility and portability.

(b) Using strategic, regional, and local forces flexibly, achieving consistency of the "three-stage" mobility and allocation.

As the supporting forces near disaster areas, regional supporting forces are important for early treatment and response, and the advantages of regional supporting forces in emergency medical rescue forces in the Yushu earthquake mainly comprise rapid mobility and allocation, as well as the ability to adapt to the high-altitude conditions. The local forces in disaster areas are mainly responsible for emergency treatment after earthquakes and emergency treatment tasks. Following the Yushu earthquake, the local emergency medical rescue forces were mainly mixed with supporting forces in the later period, which not only solved the language barrier problems for the supporting forces but also improved the utilization efficiency of the local forces. In general, the utilization of strategic regional and local emergency medical rescue forces still lacks a unified allocation principle and basis. In the future, emergency medical rescue in earthquakes, the utilization principles of emergency medical rescue forces should be established at all levels, the responsibilities and rescue needs of different levels of supporting forces should be clarified, strategic supporting forces should provide technical guidance and support, and regional supporting forces conduct relevant technological force protection or corresponding supporting protection in these regions. All types of professional forces should use utilization principles collectively: adhere to the localization management in disaster areas (according to areas of responsibility), regional protection, and determination of the scope of treatment technologies and casualty evacuation system. Combined with the "two phases and three sections" of emergency medical rescue after earthquakes, emergency medical rescue forces should be utilized in accordance with the characteristics of different periods for mobilization and allocation. Emergency rescue should fully consider the characteristics of extreme medical needs in disaster areas, mobilizing rescue forces early, adequately, efficiently, and modularly. In terms of force allocation, emergency rescue should adhere to rapid and forward allocation, establish the module allocation system during the entire process, realize the high degree of consistency between force mobility and allocation, reduce inefficient losses of force utilization, and improve the efficiency of emergency medical rescue.

(c) Emphasize construction of emergency medical rescue forces in earthquake and allocate professional forces rationally according to demands.

Trauma and crush injuries account for more than 80 % of injuries in earthquakes, significantly increasing the demand for professional surgical treatment. To continually improve the establishment of national emergency medical rescue forces, emergency medical rescue professional teams should be established for earthquakes, and the force unit should improve in line with goals of being deeper with increased structural stability and rapid mobility. Emergency medical rescue professional teams for earthquakes should be established, accumulating professional treatment experiences in emergency medicine, severe trauma treatment, and methods through daily medical practices (Xu et al. 2013; Zhang et al. 2010). Intensive daily training should be conducted for the medical unit. Various kinds of personnel in medical teams should distribute on-side first-aid training for the sick and the wounded, including ventilation, bleeding, bandaging, fixed transportation, and technical training on basic life support, so that members can skillfully use the corresponding tools and equipment, learn standard writing and transmission of injury tickets, registers, and simple cases. Members of medical teams must be aware of the treatment of common diseases in earthquakes, such as the on-site first-aid treatment for crush syndrome. Meanwhile, attention must be directed toward dealing with hypoxia syndrome in the highland plateau when conducting missions, handling heat stroke when operating at high temperatures, and dealing with frostbite when operating in cold seasons. Emphasis should be placed on the professional forces and realizing module allocation and utilization.

Professional forces should allocate according to demands. First, medical evacuation force allocation should be in accordance with on-site first aid and professional treatment and, if necessary, arrange early treatment stages. Based on localization management and requirements of regional protection, protection regions should be divided uniformly, and the scope of treatment technologies and the casualty evacuation system should be determined. Second, the health and epidemic prevention forces should be allocated based on principles of the combination of the primary and professional epidemic prevention forces and the combination of mobilized forces and regional forces.

9.2.6 *Structure of the Organization and Command of Earthquake Rescue Forces Model*

9.2.6.1 Construction of the Organization and Command of Earthquake Rescue Forces Model

Our purpose was to present behavioral modeling for some applications using autonomous agents in real environments (geographical regions) and show that this can be a useful approach for simulation of complex systems (military conflicts, urban and environmental phenomena, etc.). This case study demonstrates that effective coordination during major emergencies requires the development of a deeper, shared understanding of the incident and a high level of trust between responding organizations, both of which require effort to achieve and are difficult to support with current communications systems. Adoption of a sociotechnical systems approach during the development process may enable future communication systems to support these important social processes. Operations other than war are a real test of joint military–civilian operations and provide a practical platform for military and civilian forms of collaboration for the new era of innovation.

The basis of this research is collaborative theory, complex adaptive systems theory, multi-agent systems theory, and disaster medical rescue theory. Learning from non-warfare military action, our research group made integrated use of analytic hierarchy process, gray relational analysis, Delphi, expert survey, consulting method, and other methods used in Yushu City, Qinghai, in the Yushu earthquake medical relief operation field investigation. Meanwhile, soldiers participating in a major disaster medical rescue operation received a questionnaire survey. Based on the results of the survey data and expert advice, we defined the collaborative command of the main attributes, rules of conduct, and the trend of diversification of the operations other than war and improved the efficiency of collaborative command and effects by constructing mathematical models to describe the abstraction mechanism for collaborative command and complex process simulation software to simulate the type and extent of synergy, collaborative command efficiency, and system performance to explore a variety of factors. With regard to related theory, the study provides new tools and methods.

(a) Reduce the command hierarchy and strengthen the command coordination.
In the Yushu earthquake, medical relief work has been improved by the rule of "two level-four units," with the Joint Assembly able to achieve the integration of the military and local work modes. The rule of "two level-four units" will play an important role in the disaster medical rescue, casualty evacuation, epidemic prevention, and high-altitude disease prevention fields. The efficient emergency medical rescue cooperation among transportation, railway, civil aviation, earthquake, civil affairs, and meteorological departments reflects the efficient collaboration between health and non-health department command subjects.

(b) Shorten the emergency rescue run-in time and strengthen the communication between military and local rescue forces.
The content of the rescue mission includes the use of force, command and organization relationships, material guarantees, policy guarantee, and communication with the related national department. Improving coordination between military and civil forces and establishing efficient communication system can help to achieve higher efficiency and effectiveness during emergency medical rescue work.
(c) Strengthen the construction of the planning and legal system for emergencies.
Only strengthening construction of the legal system and perfecting various plans and laws can we respond to emergencies efficiently and minimize loss with relevant laws and regulations.

9.2.7 *The Structure of Location and Distribution of Medical Rescue Institutions Model*

9.2.7.1 Construction of Location and Distribution of Medical Rescue Institutions Model

Location means selecting the location at which one or several service facilities in a certain area allow a certain indicator to reach the optimum value. Such issues can often be encountered in the planning and construction. For choosing the dispatch districts for medical supporting institutions, location optimization model is designed to use the theoretical model and GIS to discuss the location optimization of the medical supporting institutions and provide rapid decision-making methods for medical assistance under uncertainty. The medical supporting institutions have their respective mandates, so the significance of choosing locations varies (Abolghasemi et al. 2005). The location optimization of medical supporting institutions starts from the location decision unit, which is affiliated with the "wartime deployment" problem of medical service command and securing the decision problem matrix. It focuses on the study of location optimization issues under uncertainty, through screening from the location of medical supporting institutions under emergency and wartime conditions, to select representative medical supporting institutions as model targets and conduct related studies on optimization modeling.

According to the theory of military health resource allocation, Spatial Decision Support System (SDSS) and computer software development technology, using preliminary studies of the task force as reference, this thesis builds the optimized distribution model of regional medical resources, reveals the optimized distribution configuration mechanism of regional army medical resources, proposes the optimized distribution configuration plan of regional army medical resources, and settles the reasonable distribution and utilization efficiency of army medical resources. All of these are based on medical service demand and utilization of military personnel, the status and prediction of regional military medical resource allocation, and the situation analysis of regional military medical resource distribution.

9.2.7.2 Result of the Simulation of the Model of Location and Distribution of Medical Rescue Institutions

Through analyzing the impact of medical supporting institution locations, and using Analytic Hierarchy Process to determine the weight value of each factor, the combat zone can be divided into several smaller areas based on GIS database information system. Based on the weight values of each influencing factor carried out by Analytic Hierarchy Process and using the GIS spatial analysis functions, these qualitative and quantitative factors and other relevant information in the smallest unit of an internal location in the approximate geographical location can be achieved. Then, a plurality of candidate points of the weight value information will be obtained, and through the minimum weight limit identified by the decision maker, the corresponding candidate points can be obtained. Finally, according to the minimum distance from the medical supporting institution to each object to protect, the best alternative solution is determined.

9.2.8 Structure of the "from Peacetime to Wartime in Hospital Model"

9.2.8.1 Construction of the "from Peacetime to Wartime in Hospital Model"

The research followed the ideology of "evidence-based research" to investigate the mechanism of potentiality management, capability development, and implementation of civilian hospital mobilization. Referring to Complexity Adapt System (CAS) modeling theory, the authors devised a CHM System Dynamics (SD) model with research methods especially SD modeling technique. With the SD model of the CHM system, the behavior rules were stimulated, and analog simulation of the system structure and complicated behavior were realized, thus providing a test platform for relevant policy-making. Intervening tests were then carried out on the platform to find the intervening target for improving system performance. Policy recommendations proposed to increase the capacity of CHM system provide a theoretical basis for the building of mobilization capacity.

9.2.8.2 Result of the Simulation and Intervention of the "from Peacetime to Wartime in Hospital Model"

(a) For civilian hospital mobilization, mobilization speed and mobilization cost are often the key factors.
    Speed and efficiency are remarkable features of civilian hospital hygiene mobilization, the increase of mobilization effects is largely affected by mobilization speed, and rapid mobilization has become the main form of hygiene mobilization.

(b) Modest scale of reservists is conducive to implementation of rapid mobilization.
Construction of civilian hospital mobilization focuses on strengthening the connection of mobilization in peacetime and wartime and improving the rapid response capability of mobilization. The education of necessary military medicine, military pharmacy, and military general knowledge to medical reservists in peacetime is beneficial to improve the mobilization capacity in peacetime and rapidly form effective treatment capability during the mobilization period. However, the scale of medical reservist force should not be too large or too small. If the scale of reservists is too large, it will aggravate the national burden; if the scale is too small, the reservists cannot be qualified for missions and tasks. Therefore, the scale of the medical reservist force should be moderate.

(c) A sensitive and efficient mobilization command system is a prerequisite for completion of medical mobilization tasks.
Enhancing effectiveness of organization and command mobilization is the key to improving mobilization efficiency in civilian hospitals. We should establish a scientific, rational, authoritative, and efficient organization leadership system of civilian hospital mobilization, improve the command institution that can adapt to requirements of war and crisis, and constantly improve the military and political linkage mechanism, as well as coordinate tightly, interact with supply and demand, and share resources when organizing and implementing mobilization activities.

(d) The level of compensation for mobilized medical personnel has a relatively great impact on the effect of mobilization.
Therefore, when implementing medical manpower mobilization, countries should compensate for the losses suffered by mobilized personnel when fulfilling their mobilization obligations, thus protecting the interests of mobilized personnel. Countries should ensure the protection of their income and employment status during their service, address their concerns, and provide appropriate policies to those medical institutions that actively cooperate with defense constructions in peacetime and after wars. This will undoubtedly address concerns of medical personnel and institutions, effectively improve medical personnel's enthusiasms to be involved in mobilization, and create conditions for medical personnel to fully exercise their talents to safeguard national security interests.

References

Abolghasemi H, Poorheidari G, Mehrabi A, Foroutan G. Iranian military forces in the Bam earthquake. Mil Med. 2005;170(10):859–61.

Kang P, Zhang L, Liang W, Zhu Z, Liu Y, Xu L, Yang H. Medical evacuation management and clinical characteristics of 3,255 inpatients after the 2010 Yushu earthquake in China. J Trauma Acute Care Surg. 2012;72(6):1626–33.

Liu XU, Lu Lu Zhang, Yuan Liu, Yi Zhang. Analysis and reflections on medical evacuation in Wenchuan earthquake relief. Hosp Admin J Chinese Peoples Liberation Army. 2009;16(3): 249–51.

Lulu Z, Xu L, Youping L, Yuan L, Zhipeng L, Lin J, Shen J, Xuefeng T, Yi Z, Liang W. Emergency medical rescue efforts after a major earthquake: lessons from the 2008 Wenchuan earthquake. Lancet. 2012;379(9818):853–61.

Xiang B, Cheng W, Liu J, Huang L, Li Y, Liu L. Triage of pediatric injuries after the 2008 Wen-Chuan earthquake in China. J Pediatr Surg. 2009;44(12):2273–7.

Xu L, Yuan L, Zhang L, Liang W, Zhu Z, Shen Y, Peng K, Liu Z. Mass aeromedical evacuation of patients in an emergency: experience following the 2010 Yushu earthquake. J Emerg Med. 2013;45(6):865–71.

Zhang L, Yuan L, Xu L, Yi Z. Rescue efforts management and characteristics of casualties of the Wenchuan earthquake in China. Emerg Med J. 2010;28(7):618–22.

GPSR Compliance

The European Union's (EU) General Product Safety Regulation (GPSR) is a set of rules that requires consumer products to be safe and our obligations to ensure this.

If you have any concerns about our products, you can contact us on ProductSafety@springernature.com

In case Publisher is established outside the EU, the EU authorized representative is:

Springer Nature Customer Service Center GmbH
Europaplatz 3
69115 Heidelberg, Germany

Batch number: 09223851

Printed by Printforce, the Netherlands